Study Guide to Accompany
Surgical Technology for the Surgical Technologist: A Positive Care Approach

The Association of Surgical Technologists, Inc.

Teri L. Junge, CST/CFA
Education Coordinator, Association of Surgical Technologists

DELMAR
THOMSON LEARNING

Australia • Canada • Mexico • Singapore • Spain • United Kingdom • United States

Study Guide to Accompany
Surgical Technology for the Surgical Technologist: A Positive Care Approach

Business Unit Director:
William Brottmiller

Acquisitions Editor:
Maureen Muncaster

Development Editor:
Deb Flis

Editorial Assistant:
Maria Perretta

Executive Marketing Manager:
Dawn Gerrain

Channel Manager:
Tara Carter

Executive Production Manager:
Karen Leet

Project Editor:
Mary Ellen Cox

Production Coordinator:
Barbara A. Bullock

Art/Design Coordinator:
Rich Killar, Timothy J. Conners

COPYRIGHT © 2001 by Delmar, a division of Thomson Learning, Inc. Thomson Learning™ is a trademark used herein under license.

Printed in the United States of America
1 2 3 4 5 XXX 05 04 02 01 00

For more information contact Delmar, 3 Columbia Circle, PO Box 15015, Albany, NY 12212-5015.

Or find us on the World Wide Web at http://www.delmar.com

ALL RIGHTS RESERVED. No part of this work covered by the copyright hereon may be reproduced or used in any form or by any means—graphic, electronic, or mechanical, including photocopying, recording, taping, Web distribution or information storage and retrieval systems—without written permission of the publisher.

For permission to use material from this text or product, contact us by
Tel   (800) 730-2214
Fax (800) 730-2215
www.thomsonrights.com

Library of Congress Catalog Card Number 00-020107

NOTICE TO THE READER

Publisher does not warrant or guarantee any of the products described herein or perform any independent analysis in connection with any of the product information contained herein. Publisher does not assume, and expressly disclaims, any obligation to obtain and include information other than that provided to it by the manufacturer.

The reader is expressly warned to consider and adopt all safety precautions that might be indicated by the activities herein and to avoid all potential hazards. By following the instructions contained herein, the reader willingly assumes all risks in connection with such instructions.

The Publisher makes no representation or warranties of any kind, including but not limited to, the warranties of fitness for particular purpose or merchantability, nor are any such representations implied with respect to the material set forth herein, and the publisher takes no responsibility with respect to such material. The publisher shall not be liable for any special, consequential, or exemplary damages resulting, in whole or part, from the readers' use of, or reliance upon, this material.

Table of Contents

Preface   v

■ SECTION 1
Introduction to Surgical Technology

Chapter 1
Orientation to Surgical Technology   1

Chapter 2
The Surgical Patient   5

Chapter 3
Physical Environment and Safety Standards   9

■ SECTION 2
Principles and Practice of Surgical Technology

Chapter 4
Asepsis   13

Chapter 5
General Patient Care and Safety   29

Chapter 6
Surgical Pharmacology and Anesthesia   49

Chapter 7
Instrumentation, Equipment, and Supplies   67

Chapter 8
Wound Healing, Sutures, Needles, and Stapling Devices   79

Chapter 9
The Surgical Technologist in the Scrub Role (Case Management)   91

■ SECTION 3
Surgical Procedures

Chapter 10
Diagnostic Procedures   133

Chapter 11
General Surgery   147

Chapter 12
Obstetric and Gynecologic Surgery   159

Chapter 13
Ophthalmic Surgery   171

Chapter 14
Otorhinolaryngologic Surgery   185

Chapter 15
Oral and Maxillofacial Surgery   199

Chapter 16
Plastic and Reconstructive Surgery   213

Chapter 17
Genitourinary Surgery   227

Chapter 18
Orthopedic Surgery   243

Chapter 19
Cardiothoracic Surgery   259

Chapter 20
Peripheral Vascular Surgery   275

Chapter 21
Neurosurgery   291

PREFACE

TO THE SURGICAL TECHNOLOGY STUDENT

The textbook *Surgical Technology for the Surgical Technologist: A Positive Care Approach* defines the cognitive model necessary for the surgical technologist to function effectively and provides an innovative approach for learning the role of the surgical technologist while focusing on the knowledge and skills that will be required. This model leads the way for the surgical technology student to remember the pertinent information using the predictive model: *A Positive Care Approach*. Because the text was written by surgical technologists and surgical technology educators, the needs of the student have been considered throughout the process. The graduate of a CAAHEP (Commission on Accreditation of Allied Health Education Programs) accredited surgical technology program will meet the eligibility requirements of the LCC-ST (Liaison Council on Certification for the Surgical Technologist) to sit for the national certifying examination for the surgical technologist.

The basic steps of the cognitive process for the surgical technologist are defined by Bob Caruthers, CST, PhD, Deputy Director, Association of Surgical Technologists.

The surgical technologist:

- has a mental image of normal anatomy
- makes a mental comparison of the idealized anatomy with the actual anatomy of a specific patient
- knows an idealized operative procedure used to correct the pathologic condition
- makes a mental comparison of the idealized procedure with the actual procedure being performed
- allows for a particular surgeon's variations to the idealized procedure
- allows for variances in anatomy, pathology, and surgeons' responses to the variances
- predicts and prepares to meet the needs of the surgeon and surgical patient prior to verbalization of the need

To facilitate the learning process, *Surgical Technology for the Surgical Technologist: A Positive Care Approach* has been divided into two major sections. These divisions correspond to the *A Positive Care Approach* and are represented by the A POSitive and CARE acronyms. The first nine chapters are related to the CARE acronym. The CARE division itself is divided into two sections: (1) Introduction to Surgical Technology, and (2) Principles and Practice of Surgical Technology. The last twelve chapters relate to the A POSitive acronym; a brief introduction to diagnostics is followed by chapters focusing on operative procedures for various surgical specialties.

What is the A Positive Care Approach? It is a systematic approach to surgical problem solving focused on the ability of the surgical technologist to predict the needs of the surgeon and patient. The A Positive Care Approach uses two simple memory tools for systematic problem solving.

The CARE division will establish a broad context in which the instructor will help the student place the more specific technical information that dominates surgical technology. Introductory and foundational information is learned using the CARE approach, which is intended to serve as a reminder to the surgical technologist that all activities affect the care given to the patient. The student should be aware that the highly variable topics of the first nine, or non-procedural, chapters of the text do not allow a simple one-to-one correlation of the CARE memory tool, rather it is a conceptual tool intended to help organize the information:

C Care directed toward the patient and/or surgical team

A Aseptic principles and practice of sterile technique

R Role of the surgical technologist

E Environmental awareness and concern

The A POSitive division relates directly to the final twelve, or procedural, chapters with CARE as the underlying theme. The surgical procedures are presented by surgical specialty using the illustrative procedure format. The illustrative procedure format is based on the concept that one procedure can highlight several important steps that are repeated in related procedures. Rather than presenting many procedures with brief outlines of the steps, fewer procedures are presented in detail, thus allowing the surgical technologist to predict the necessary preparation and action to be taken. The A POSitive approach does allow the one-to-one correlation of the procedural chapter objectives and should be used to reinforce every surgical procedure encountered by the student:

A Anatomy

P Pathology

O Operative Procedure

S Specific Variations

In this Study Guide we will provide you with learning concepts and tools and a way to use them to enhance your education.

The authors of *Surgical Technology for the Surgical Technologist: A Positive Care Approach* wish you success in your endeavor to become a Certified Surgical Technologist (CST)!

Orientation to Surgical Technology

CHAPTER 1

OBJECTIVES

After studying this chapter, the reader should be able to:

C 1. Identify and demonstrate principles of communication in the surgical setting.

A 2. (No objectives focused on asepsis in this chapter; however, the student should demonstrate an awareness that the principles of asepsis are a vital component of the surgical technologist's role in surgical patient care.)

R 3. Trace the historical development of surgery and surgical technology.

4. Identify members of the surgical team and their roles.

5. Identify the various roles of the surgical technologist.

6. Identify and interpret a job description for the surgical technologist.

E 7. Identify different types of health care facilities.

8. Describe a typical hospital organizational structure.

9. Identify hospital departments and their relationships to surgical services.

CHAPTER 1

■ Key Terms

Define the following:

1. Acronym _____
   _____

2. Ambulatory Surgical Facility _____
   _____

3. ARC-ST _____
   _____

4. AST _____
   _____

5. Circulator _____
   _____

6. Competency _____
   _____

7. Core Curriculum _____
   _____

8. DO _____
   _____

9. Elective _____
   _____

10. Emergent _____
    _____

11. Fiscal _____
    _____

12. HMO _____
    _____

13. Intraoperative _____
    _____

14. JCAHO _____
    _____

15. LCC-ST _____
    _____

16. Optional _____
    _____

17. Pasteur _____
    _____

18. Postoperative _____
    _____

19. Preceptor _____
    _____

20. Preoperative _____
    _____

21. Professional _____
    _____

22. Proprietary _____
    _____

23. STSR1 _____
    _____

24. Urgent _____
    _____

25. Vesalius _____
    _____

Case Studies

☐ CASE STUDY 1

Rodrigo is a 57-year-old male who was admitted to the ED following an automobile accident. Rodrigo was driving a delivery van that was struck head-on by another vehicle. Rodrigo has severe injuries to both lower extremities: (1) closed femur fracture of the left leg and (2) open fracture of the right tibia and fibula with near amputation. A chest tube was inserted upon arrival in the ED. Rodrigo is neurologically intact. He is now scheduled for surgery on his legs.

1. This case represents what category of surgical intervention? _____

2. What is the difference between emergent and urgent surgical intervention? _____

3. What is elective surgery? _____

4. Is elective surgical intervention the same thing as "minor" surgery? _____

CHAPTER 1

☐ CASE STUDY 2

Kathleen is a 15-year-old female who has been admitted to the hospital for surgery to correct a condition called scoliosis, an abnormal lateral curvature of the spine. This surgical intervention requires a lengthy incision and dissection of spinal muscles. It runs the risk of considerable blood loss and damage to spinal nerves. Distraction rods are placed to help straighten the spine, and bone grafting is required.

1. Intraoperative X-rays are required. Who would perform these, and what department of the hospital would employ them? _____

2. Blood loss may be countered by filtering the patient's blood and returning it to her. Who would perform this activity? _____

3. Patients undergoing spinal surgery are often monitored for changes in electrical conduction to the lower extremities. Who would perform this task? _____

4. To whom would blood samples be taken in order to check for hematocrit and hemoglobin counts during the operative procedure? _____

5. An upper body cast may be applied several days postoperatively. Who would assist the surgeon in this task? _____

The Surgical Patient

CHAPTER 2

OBJECTIVES

After studying this chapter, the reader should be able to:

C 1. Assess the patient's response to illness and hospitalization.
2. Distinguish and assess the physical, spiritual, and psychological needs of a patient.
3. Distinguish and assess cultural and religious influences on the surgical patient.
4. Identify and discuss the rights of the health care consumer.
5. Describe the general needs associated with special populations of surgical patients.

A 6. Demonstrate awareness that all surgical patients have the right to the highest standards and practices in asepsis.

R 7. Describe the process used to obtain an informed consent for surgical treatment and discuss the legal restrictions involved.

E 8. Discuss the principle of documentation in the health care environment.
9. Define and interpret ethical, moral, and legal responsibilities.
10. Demonstrate an understanding of common legal terms used in the health care environment.

CHAPTER 2

■ Key Terms

Define the following:

1. Accountability _____
   _____

2. Accreditation _____
   _____

3. *aeger primo* _____
   _____

4. Benign _____
   _____

5. Consent _____
   _____

6. Credential _____
   _____

7. Disease _____
   _____

8. Emancipated Minor _____
   _____

9. Ethics _____
   _____

10. Geriatrics _____
    _____

11. HIV _____
    _____

12. Iatrogenic _____
    _____

13. Incident Report _____
    _____

14. Malignant _____
    _____

15. Maslow's Hierarchy of Needs _____
    _____

16. Negligence _____
    _____

17. Neonate _____
    _____

18. Neoplasm _____
    _____

19. Patient _____
    _____

20. Patient's Bill of Rights _____
    _____

21. Physical Need _____
    _____

22. Prioritize _____
    _____

23. Psychological Need _____
    _____

24. Social Need _____
    _____

25. Spiritual Need _____
    _____

Case Studies

CASE STUDY 1

Mollie is a 9-year-old female who was admitted to the hospital following a seizure on the playground at school. She has been diagnosed with a cerebral arteriovenous malformation. A craniotomy with attendant clipping and removal of the AVM has been proposed. Mollie is in a foster home. Her biological parents are both dead.

1. What is needed for a valid consent for surgery in this case? _____

2. Who can give consent in this case? _____

3. Can the surgical intervention be refused? _____

CASE STUDY 2

Harold is still a relatively new surgical technologist. Since passing the national certification examination, he has been working in a large teaching hospital. He loves the work and being at a hospital "on the cutting edge." He is surprised to find out that several of the staff members do not think they should be performing some of the procedures they do. They feel that it is like experimenting on human beings.

1. Do you believe health care professionals are required to do everything necessary to save and prolong human life? _____

continues

CASE STUDY 2 (continued)

2. What is more important: quality or quantity of life? How do you know what quality is? _____

3. Is there such a thing as a "right to die?" _____

4. Does a health care professional have the right to refuse to participate in approved procedures? _____

CHAPTER 3

Physical Environment and Safety Standards

OBJECTIVES

After studying this chapter, the reader should be able to:

C 1. Identify and describe hazards to the patient in the operative environment.

2. Identify support services that work with the OR team in the care of the patient.

A 3. Understand the type of air-handling system required in the OR and the temperature and humidity required to maintain a sterile field.

4. Identify cleaning procedures, traffic patterns, and routines required in the operative environment.

R 5. Identify the role of the surgical technologist in the protection of self, patients, and others from hazards in the operative environment.

E 6. Identify the design types of the OR.

7. Identify hospital departments that relate to surgical services.

8. Understand the working environment of the OR.

9. Identify the physical components of the OR.

Key Terms

Define the following:

1. Airborne _____

2. Back Table _____

3. Decontamination _____

4. Electrosurgical Unit _____

5. Ergonomics _____

6. Hamper _____

7. HEPA Filter _____

8. Hopper _____

9. Hypothermia _____

10. Ionizing Radiation _____

11. Laminar Flow _____

12. Mayo Stand _____

13. Methyl Methacrylate _____

14. OSHA _____

15. Pathology Department _____

16. Perfusionist _____

17. Plume _____

18. Postanesthesia Care Unit _____

19. PPE _____

20. Prophylaxis _____

21. Restricted Area _____

22. SSI _____

23. Standard Precautions _____

24. Suction Outlet _____

25. Triboelectrification _____

Case Studies

CASE STUDY 1

Eloise is preparing to scrub for an open reduction internal fixation (ORIF) of a tibial plateau fracture. Intraoperative X-rays will be taken.

1. What special communications with other departments/personnel will be necessary prior to this procedure? _____
_____
_____
_____
_____

2. Will Eloise need to wear any personal protective equipment (PPE) for this procedure? _____
_____
_____
_____
_____

3. Will the patient require any safety equipment during the procedure? _____
_____
_____
_____
_____

4. The presence of an X-ray tech in the room presents a special situation. What responsibility does Eloise have during this time? _____
_____
_____
_____
_____

CHAPTER 3

☐ CASE STUDY 2

Today is Saturday; the staff in the operating room is limited. Marcus has been assigned to a femoro-popliteal bypass surgery that could take six to eight hours. During the week, the OR staff can expect to be relieved for lunch, but today Marcus knows that is unlikely to happen.

1. What can Marcus do in advance to physically prepare himself for this lengthy procedure? _____

   _____
   _____
   _____
   _____

2. Are there any tips that you can give Marcus to reduce the strain on his body while the case is in progress? _____

   _____
   _____
   _____
   _____

Asepsis

CHAPTER 4

OBJECTIVES

After studying this chapter, the reader should be able to:

C 1. Discuss the relationship between the Principles of Asepsis and the Practice of Sterile Technique to surgical patient care.

2. Define and discuss the concept of surgical conscience.

A 3. Discuss the principles of asepsis.

4. Define the terms related to asepsis.

5. Discuss the practices related to the principles of asepsis.

6. Identify the principles and procedures related to disinfection and sterilization.

R 7. Demonstrate competency related to the practice of sterile technique.

8. Demonstrate competency in the procedures related to disinfection and sterilization.

E 9. Discuss the surgical environment and the application of the principles of asepsis to the environment.

CHAPTER 4

■ Key Terms

Define the following:

1. Asepsis _____

2. Bioburden _____

3. Biological Indicator _____

4. Bowie-Dick Test _____

5. Chelation _____

6. Chemical Indicator _____

7. Colonization _____

8. Contaminated _____

9. Emulsification _____

10. Endoscope _____

11. Event-Related Sterility _____

12. Flash Sterilization _____

13. Immersion _____

14. Integrity _____

15. Intermediate Disinfection _____

16. Julian Date _____

17. Lister _____

18. Lumen _____

19. Pathogen _____

20. Permeability _____

21. Sterile _____

22. Sterile Technique _____

23. Subungual _____

24. Surgical Conscience _____

25. Ultrasonic Washer _____

Case Studies

CASE STUDY 1

Brittney telephoned her physician to report that she is experiencing a fever of 101°F seven days following her laparoscopic tubal ligation. She also states that she is experiencing urinary frequency and burning during urination. The physician suspects that Brittney may be suffering from a urinary tract infection because of the catheter that was used to empty her bladder during the surgical procedure. The physician has asked Brittney to schedule an appointment later in the day so that he may examine her and obtain a "clean catch" urine sample.

1. Would Brittney's infection be considered a surgical site infection (SSI)? If not, what type of infection is it?

   _____
   _____
   _____
   _____

2. What is the most likely reason that Brittney is suffering from an infection?

   _____
   _____
   _____
   _____
   _____

CASE STUDY 2

Ned is preparing the operating room for an emergency procedure. He is rushing because he knows that the patient will soon be brought into the room and he may not have time to complete his preparations. Ned is opening the final item; just as he is about to place the item on the back table, he notices a small hole in the wrapper.

1. What moral/ethical concept will Ned use to make the "right" decision?

   _____
   _____
   _____
   _____

2. What are Ned's options, and what is the best choice?

   _____

(continues)

CASE STUDY 2 (continued)

3. If Ned makes the wrong choice, what possible impact could this have on the patient?

Skill Assessment 4-1

OR Attire

Student Name _____ Date _____

Instructor _____

Procedural Step	Adequate	Needs Review
1. Student is able to state purpose for wearing proper OR attire		
2. Student is able to state situations when variations in OR attire may occur		
3. Student is able to state when OR attire is to be worn		
4. Scrub suit		
5. No jewelry		
6. No cosmetics		
7. Hair cover		
8. Identification		
9. Radiation monitoring device		
10. Shoes appropriate to OR		
11. Shoe covers		
12. Mask		
13. Eyewear		

Comments _____
_____
_____
_____

Asepsis 19

Skill Assessment 4-2

Basic Handwash

Student Name _____ Date _____

Instructor _____

Procedural Step	Adequate	Needs Review
1. Student is able to state purpose of handwash		
2. Student is able to state circumstances when a handwash is necessary		
3. Equipment and supplies are assembled		
4. Jewelry removed		
5. Turn on faucet		
6. Inspect hands and wrists		
7. Wet hands and wrists		
8. Apply soap		
9. Lather		
10. Interlace fingers		
11. Use nail cleaner/brush (if necessary)		
12. Handwash is of appropriate duration		
13. All surfaces cleaned		
14. Rinse		
15. Turn off water		
16. Dry		
17. Discard towel(s)		

Comments _____

_____

_____

Asepsis 21

Skill Assessment 4-3

Packaging Technique – Wrap
(Envelope Fold)

Student Name _____ Date _____

Instructor _____

Procedural Step	Adequate	Needs Review
1. Student is able to state purpose for envelope-style wrap		
2. Appropriate attire		
3. Wash hands (Standard Precautions)		
4. Equipment and supplies assembled		
5. Orient wrap material on suitable surface		
6. Place item to be wrapped on wrapper		
7. Insert internal indicator		
8. Fold first flap		
9. Fold second (left) flap		
10. Fold third (right) flap		
11. Fold fourth flap		
12. Apply second wrapper (if necessary)		
13. Secure final flap		
14. Label for processing		
15. Place in designated area		
16. Proceed with other tasks		

Comments _____
_____
_____
_____

Skill Assessment 4-4

Packaging Technique – Wrap
(Square Fold)

Student Name _____ Date _____

Instructor _____

Procedural Step	Adequate	Needs Review
1. Student is able to state purpose for square-style wrap		
2. Appropriate attire		
3. Wash hands (Standard Precautions)		
4. Equipment and supplies assembled		
5. Orient wrap material on suitable surface		
6. Place item to be wrapped on wrapper		
7. Insert internal indicator		
8. Fold first flap		
9. Fold second flap		
10. Fold third flap		
11. Fold final flap		
12. Apply second wrapper (if necessary)		
13. Secure final flap		
14. Label for processing		
15. Place in designated area		
16. Proceed with other tasks		

Comments _____
_____
_____
_____

Skill Assessment 4-5

Packaging Technique – Peel Pack

Student Name _____ Date _____

Instructor _____

Procedural Step	Adequate	Needs Review
1. Student is able to state purpose for peel pack-style package		
2. Appropriate attire		
3. Wash hands (Standard Precautions)		
4. Equipment and supplies assembled		
5. Place item(s) in pouch		
6. Seal pouch		
7. Double package (if necessary)		
8. Label for processing		
9. Place in designated area		
10. Proceed with other tasks		

Comments _____

_____

_____

_____

Skill Assessment 4-6

Packaging Technique – Container System

Student Name _____ Date _____

Instructor _____

Procedural Step	Adequate	Needs Review
1. Student is able to state purpose for container-style package		
2. Appropriate attire		
3. Wash hands (Standard Precautions)		
4. Equipment and supplies assembled		
5. Prepare container		
6. Place instrument set in basket		
7. Place basket in container		
8. Place lid and seal		
9. Label for processing		
10. Place in designated area		
11. Proceed with other tasks		

Comments _____

_____

_____

_____

CHAPTER 5

General Patient Care and Safety

OBJECTIVES

After studying this chapter, the reader should be able to:

C 1. Demonstrate an understanding of the process used to obtain an informed consent for a surgical procedure or treatment.
2. Describe preoperative routines.
3. Identify, describe, and demonstrate the principles of transportation of the surgical patient.
4. Discuss, demonstrate, and apply the principles of surgical positioning.
5. Understand the methods of preparation of the operative site for surgery.
6. Describe the application of thermoregulatory devices.
7. Explain the principles and demonstrate the taking and recording of vital signs.
8. Explain the principles of urinary catheterization and demonstrate the procedure.

A 9. Describe how the principles of operative site preparation and urinary catheterization are related both to patient care and to asepsis.

R 10. Discuss methods of hemostasis and blood replacement and demonstrate the preparation and use of appropriate agents or devices.
11. Identify developing emergency situations, initiate appropriate action, and assist in treatment of the patient.
12. Discuss methods and types of documentation used in the OR.

E 13. Discuss the relationship between patient safety and the surgical environment.

CHAPTER 5

■ Key Terms

Define the following:

1. Apical Pulse _____

2. Autologous _____

3. Cardiac Dysrhythmia _____

4. Catheterization _____

5. CPR _____

6. Dyspnea _____

7. Hemolysis _____

8. Hemostasis _____

9. Hemostat _____

10. Homeostasis _____

11. Homologous _____

12. Hypertension _____

13. Informed Consent _____

14. Laser _____

15. NPO _____

16. Prep _____

17. Prone _____

18. Pulse Oximeter _____

19. Rh Factor _____

20. Sedation _____

21. Shock _____

22. Suction _____

23. Supine _____

24. Tourniquet _____

25. Vital Signs _____

Case Studies

CASE STUDY 1

Viorel is a 10-year-old male who has been adopted. He is scheduled for a right inguinal herniorrhaphy.

1. Who has the authority to sign Viorel's operative consent?

2. In what position will Viorel be placed for the herniorrhaphy?

3. Describe the anatomical area that will be prepped.

4. Are any special considerations necesssary to accommodate Viorel's age?

CASE STUDY 2

After Virginia-May was placed on the operating table, it was discovered that her surgeon would be delayed by approximately fifteen minutes. Virginia-May is 67 years old and is scheduled for a vaginal hysterectomy. She is very apprehensive.

(continues)

CHAPTER 5

☐ CASE STUDY 2 (continued)

1. What steps can be taken to help Virginia-May feel more comfortable?

   _____
   _____
   _____
   _____

2. Should the operating team continue with the preparations? For example, should she be anesthetized and positioned?

   _____
   _____
   _____
   _____

Skill Assessment 5-1

Vital Signs – Temperature

Student Name _____ Date _____

Instructor _____

Procedural Step	Adequate	Needs Review
1. Student is able to state purpose for temperature monitoring		
2. Wash hands (Standard Precautions)		
3. Equipment and supplies are assembled		
4. Equipment prepared		
5. Identify patient, self, and explain procedure (if applicable)		
6. Position patient (if necessary)		
7. Place temperature probe		
8. Probe remains in position for prescribed amount of time		
9. Hold temperature probe in place (if necessary)		
10. Carefully remove temperature probe		
11. Read thermometer		
12. Wash hands (Standard Precautions)		
13. Record or report findings		
14. Care for equipment as needed		

Comments _____

_____

_____

General Patient Care and Safety 35

Skill Assessment 5-2

Vital Signs – Pulse

Student Name _____ Date _____

Instructor _____

Procedural Step	Adequate	Needs Review
1. Student is able to state purpose for pulse measurement		
2. Wash hands (Standard Precautions)		
3. Equipment and supplies are assembled		
4. Identify patient, self, and explain procedure (if applicable)		
5. Position patient (if necessary)		
6. Locate site		
7. Compress artery (or listen with stethoscope)		
8. Note time		
9. Count pulse rate and note rhythm, volume, and condition of the arterial wall		
10. Wash hands (Standard Precautions)		
11. Record or report findings		
12. Care for equipment as needed		

Comments _____

_____

_____

_____

Skill Assessment 5-3

Vital Signs – Respiration

Student Name _____ Date _____

Instructor _____

Procedural Step	Adequate	Needs Review
1. Student is able to state purpose of respiration monitoring		
2. Student is able to state normal respiration values, identify an abnormality, and explain the implications of an abnormality		
3. Wash hands (Standard Precautions)		
4. Equipment and supplies are assembled		
5. Identify patient, self, and explain procedure (if applicable)		
6. Position patient (if necessary)		
7. Obtain respiratory rate, depth, rhythm, and breath sounds		
8. Wash hands (Standard Precautions, if necessary)		
9. Record or report findings		
10. Care for equipment as needed		

Comments _____
_____
_____
_____

Skill Assessment 5-4

Vital Signs – Blood Pressure

Student Name _____ Date _____

Instructor _____

Procedural Step	Adequate	Needs Review
1. Student is able to state purpose for blood pressure monitoring		
2. Student is able to state normal blood pressure values, identify an abnormality, and explain the implications of an abnormality		
3. Wash hands (Standard Precautions)		
4. Equipment and supplies are assembled		
5. Identify patient, self, and explain procedure (if applicable)		
6. Position patient and expose site (if necessary)		
7. Apply blood pressure cuff		
8. Place stethoscope		
9. Inflate blood pressure cuff		
10. Deflate blood pressure cuff slowly, while listening for Korotkoff's sounds		
11. Continue deflation of blood pressure cuff. Continue to note sounds		
12. Complete deflation of cuff and remove cuff (if situation allows)		
13. Wash hands (Standard Precautions)		
14. Record or report findings		
15. Care for equipment as needed		

Comments _____
_____
_____
_____

Skill Assessment 5-5

Glove Oneself – Open Glove Technique
(Not Recommended When Wearing a Sterile Gown)

Student Name _____ Date _____

Instructor _____

Procedural Step	Adequate	Needs Review
1. Student is able to state purpose for application of sterile gloves		
2. Student is able to give several examples of situations in which the open glove technique will be necessary		
3. Wash hands (Standard Precautions)		
4. Equipment and supplies are assembled		
5. Remove outer wrapper		
6. Open inner wrapper		
7. Secure first glove from wrapper		
8. Apply first glove		
9. Secure second glove from wrapper		
10. Apply second glove		
11. Keep gloved hands sterile		

Comments _____
_____
_____
_____

Skill Assessment 5-6

Remove Soiled Gloves

Student Name _____ Date _____

Instructor _____

Procedural Step	Adequate	Needs Review
1. Student is able to state purpose for using correct glove removal technique		
2. Student is able to give examples of several situations in which this technique will be employed		
3. Equipment and supplies are assembled		
4. Grasp palm of glove to be removed first with opposite hand		
5. Remove first glove		
6. Keep removed glove in hand that remains gloved		
7. Begin to remove second glove		
8. Contain first glove inside of inverted second glove		
9. Finish removal of second glove		
10. Properly dispose of gloves		
11. Wash hands (Standard Precautions)		

Comments _____
_____
_____
_____

Skill Assessment 5-7

Urinary Catheterization
(Male or Female)

Student Name _____ Date _____

Instructor _____

Procedural Step	Adequate	Needs Review
1. Student is able to define urinary catheterization		
2. Student is able to state purpose for urinary catheterization		
3. Student is able to identify several situations in which urinary catheterization will be needed		
4. Student is able to identify different types of equipment that may be needed and state examples of when each may be used		
5. Wash hands (Standard Precautions)		
6. Equipment and supplies are assembled		
7. Identify patient, self, and explain procedure (if applicable)		
8. Position and expose patient		
9. Provide adequate lighting		
10. Remove protective cover and open catheter kit		
11. Don sterile gloves		
12. Organize supplies within sterile field		
13. Apply sterile drapes		
14. Cleanse meatus		
15. Insert catheter		
16. Inflate balloon		
17. Position catheter		
18. Care for patient and supplies as needed		
19. Wash hands (Standard Precautions)		
20. Document procedure		

Comments _____

_____

_____

_____

Skill Assessment 5-8

Skin Prep

Student Name _____ Date _____

Instructor _____

Procedural Step	Adequate	Needs Review
1. Student is able to define surgical skin prep		
2. Student is able to state purpose for surgical skin prep		
3. Student is able to identify several situations that will require skin prep		
4. Student is able to identify different types of equipment and supplies that may be needed		
5. Wash hands (Standard Precautions)		
6. Equipment and supplies are assembled		
7. Identify patient, self, and explain procedure (if applicable)		
8. Position and expose patient		
9. Provide adequate lighting		
10. Open prep set		
11. Don sterile gloves		
12. Organize supplies within sterile field		
13. Apply sterile drapes		
14. Apply antiseptic solution to patient's skin		
15. Dry		
16. Apply "paint"		
17. Care for patient and supplies as needed		
18. Wash hands (Standard Precautions)		
19. Document procedure		

Comments _____

_____

_____

_____

CHAPTER 6

Surgical Pharmacology and Anesthesia

OBJECTIVES

After studying this chapter, the reader should be able to:

C 1. Define general terminology and abbreviations associated with pharmacology and anesthesia.

2. Describe the action, uses, and modes of administration of drugs and anesthetic agents used in the care of the surgical patient.

3. Describe the side effects and contraindications for use for drugs and anesthetic agents.

4. Describe the factors that influence anesthesia selection for individual patients.

A 5. Demonstrate safe practice in transferring drugs and solutions from the nonsterile area to the sterile field.

6. Demonstrate the procedure for identifying a drug or solution on the sterile field.

7. Explain how sterile technique is used in relation to certain anesthesia procedures.

R 8. Convert equivalents from one system to another and accurately identify, mix, and measure drugs for patient use.

9. Explain the roles of the STSR and circulator during the administration of anesthesia.

E 10. Discuss care and precautions in identifying drugs and solutions in the OR.

11. List the equipment used as an adjunct to anesthesia.

CHAPTER 6

■ Key Terms

Define the following:

1. Agonist _____

2. Amnesia _____

3. Anaphylaxis _____

4. Anesthesia _____

5. Antagonist _____

6. Antimuscarinic _____

7. Aspiration _____

8. Biotechnology _____

9. Buccal _____

10. Capnography _____

11. Contraindication _____

12. Doppler _____

13. Drug _____

14. Generic _____

15. Homeostasis _____

16. Hypnosis _____

17. Iatrogenic _____

18. Indication _____

19. Induction _____

20. Intra-articular _____

21. Laryngospasm _____

22. NPO _____

23. PACU _____

24. Parenteral _____

25. Pharmacodynamics _____

26. Pharmacokinetics _____

27. Pharmacology _____

28. Prophylaxis _____

29. Topical _____

30. Volatile Agents _____

Exercise A – Start and Maintain a Medication File

The student will keep an ongoing file of medications commonly used showing: Name of Drug – Generic Name (Trade Name), Drug Classification, Kinetics (drug action), Route(s) of Administration, Contraindications, and Possible Iatrogenic, Adverse, or Idiosyncratic Reactions. (Index Cards work well for this exercise.)

Additionally, the instructor may have the student include on the back of the card: Usual Dosages, Special Administration and Storage Instructions, Antagonist, Drug Interactions, Overdose Symptoms and Management, and Typical Onset, Peak Effect, and Duration Times.

Sample:

front

Drug Name:

Drug Classification:

Drug Action:

Route(s) of Administration:

Possible Iatrogenic, Adverse, or Idiosyncratic Reactions:

Contraindications:

back

Antagonist:

Special Administration and Storage Instructions:

Usual Dosages:

Onset:

Peak Effect:

Preoperatively:

Duration Time:

Pain Management:

Drug Interactions:

MAO Inhibitors:

Overdose Symptoms:

Overdose Management:

Exercise B – Metric Conversions

Perform the following computations and exercises. Refer to Table 6-3 in the textbook if necessary.

1. Identify the following abbreviations.

    A. C _____

    B. m _____

    C. kg _____

    D. L _____

    E. µl _____

    F. F _____

    G. mm _____

    H. mg _____

    I. g _____

    J. dl _____

    K. m _____

    L. µg _____

    M. ml _____

    N. cm _____

    O. km _____

    P. cc _____

2. Calculate the following weight conversions.

    A. 14 lb = _____ kg

    B. 123 lb = _____ kg

    C. 46 kg = _____ lb

    D. 78 kg = _____ lb

    E. 4000 g = _____ kg

    F. 4000 g = _____ lb

    G. 1 g = _____ mg

    H. 2000 mg = _____ oz

    I. 4 oz = _____ g

    J. 114 g = _____ mg

3. Calculate the following length conversions.

    A. 1 km = _____ m

    B. 1000 m = _____ miles

    C. 4 miles = _____ km

    D. 2 m = _____ inches

    E. 17 inches = _____ cm

    F. 30 mm = _____ inches

    G. 100 cm = _____ inches

    H. 1 inch = _____ cm

    I. 1 inch = _____ mm

    J. 1 yard = _____ cm

4. Calculate the following volume conversions.

    A. 1 ml = _____ cc

    B. 4 cc = _____ ml

    C. 2 oz = _____ cc

    D. 5 liters = _____ cc

    E. 1 dl = _____ ml

    F. 0.102 oz = _____ ml

    G. 500 cc = _____ L

    H. 0.75 L = _____ cc

    I. 0.034 oz = _____ cc

    J. 12 ml = _____ oz

5. Calculate the following temperature conversions.

    A. 4°C = _____ F

    B. 32°F = _____ C

    C. 98.6°F = _____ C

    D. 0°F = _____ C

    E. 18°C = _____ F

    F. 101°F = _____ C

    G. 104°F = _____ C

    H. 212°F = _____ C

I. 81°C = _____ F

J. 91.4°F = _____ C

■ Exercise C – Identification

1. The trade names for several commonly used medications are listed. Provide the generic name.

   A. Ancef _____
   B. Anectine _____
   C. Coumadin _____
   D. Dantrium _____
   E. Decadron _____
   F. Demerol _____
   G. Forane _____
   H. Gelfoam _____
   I. Humulin _____
   J. Kantrex _____
   K. Lasix _____
   L. Marcaine _____
   M. Miochol _____
   N. Narcan _____
   O. Pitocin _____
   P. Robinul _____
   Q. Sublimaze _____
   R. Tagamet _____
   S. Toradol _____
   T. Tracrium _____
   U. Tylenol _____
   V. Valium _____
   W. Versed _____
   X. Wydase _____

2. Identify the components of the syringe shown in Figure 6-1.

Figure 6-1

A. _____ D. _____
B. _____ E. _____
C. _____

3. Identify the components of the needle shown in Figure 6-2.

Figure 6-2

A. _____ D. _____
B. _____ E. _____
C. _____ F. _____

■ Exercise D – CARE for Your Patient

Make these practical decisions.

Figure 6-3 (Courtesy of the Upjohn Company)

54 CHAPTER 6

1. The physician has ordered 5,000 units of heparin. What volume of heparin will be needed? Use the medication label pictured in Figure 6-3 to determine your answer. _____
   _____
   _____

2. From which source is heparin derived? _____
   _____

3. The surgeon preference card calls for topical thrombin. Where will the STSR initially locate the medication? _____
   _____

Figure 6-4 (Courtesy of Jones Pharma)

4. In which drug form is topical thrombin manufactured? _____
   _____

5. What must be done to prepare the medication for use? _____
   _____

6. What unit of measure is used to determine the dosage of topical thrombin? Use the medication label pictured in Figure 6-4 to determine your answer. _____
   _____

7. The physician has ordered 100,000 units of bacitracin, diluted in 1,000 cc of saline, for irrigation of the abdominal cavity. How many vials of bacitracin will be needed? Use the medication label pictured in Figure 6-5 to determine your answer. _____
   _____

8. In which drug form is bacitracin manufactured?
   _____

Figure 6-5 (Courtesy of Pharma-Tek, Inc.)

9. What must be done to prepare bacitracin for use? _____
   _____

10. How will the bacitracin/saline solution be introduced into the abdominal cavity? What supplies will be necessary? _____
    _____

11. Cocaine HCl 4% has been ordered as a local anesthetic for a patient having nasal surgery. Will the cocaine be injected? _____
    _____

12. What is the drug classification for cocaine? _____
    _____

13. If any cocaine remains at the end of the procedure, is any special procedure necessary to ensure proper disposal? Why? _____
    _____

Figure 6-6 (Courtesy of Apothecon)

14. The physician preference card calls for 1 g of kanamycin. How many vials of kanamycin will be needed? Use the medication label in Figure 6-6 to determine your answer. _____

15. What is the drug classification for kanamycin? _____

16. For what purpose would kanamycin be ordered? _____

17. What is the drug classification for oxytocin? _____

18. In what situation(s) in the operating room is the use of oxytocin indicated? _____

19. The surgeon has requested that the STSR have 20 units of oxytocin available on the sterile field. How many vials will be necessary? Use the medication label in Figure 6-7 to determine your answer. _____

Figure 6-7 (Courtesy of Novartis Pharmaceuticals Corp.)

SANDOZ
Syntocinon®
(oxytocin)
injection, USP

10 USP (1 mL ampul)
1 mL contains 10
USP or International
Units of oxytocin
FOR I.M. OR I.V. USE
Sandoz
East Hanover, NJ
22188002

20. Via which route(s) is oxytocin administered? _____

■ Case Studies

☐ CASE STUDY 1

Amanda, a 22-month-old female, is scheduled to have a percutaneous liver biopsy under general anesthesia at 7:30 AM. Her mother states that she has been NPO since last evening when she drank a bottle of 2% milk about 8:00 PM.

1. Why will Amanda be having a general anesthetic?

2. Has Amanda been NPO for an adequate amount of time?

(continues)

CASE STUDY 1 (continued)

3. How will the anesthetist determine the approximate size of Amanda's trachea?

4. How are pediatric drug dosages calculated?

5. What special anesthesia equipment, if any, will be needed to care for Amanda?

CASE STUDY 2

Tony, an 86-year-old male, is scheduled for a ventral herniorrhaphy with general anesthesia. An IV line has been inserted in Tony's left forearm. You have been asked to assist the anesthesiologist and the circulator as they position Tony on the operating table and apply the devices that will be used to monitor his condition while he is anesthetized.

1. Will Tony's position remain the same for his anesthetic administration and the procedure? What position(s) will be necessary?

(continues)

CASE STUDY 2 (continued)

2. Place the following monitors and safety devices on Tony. Indicate placement by writing the corresponding letters on the diagram of Tony (Figure 6-8). Provide your rationale for each placement decision.

Figure 6-8

A. IV - _____

B. Thermometer - _____

C. Blood Pressure Cuff - _____

D. Pulse Oximeter - _____

E. Safety Strap - _____

F. Electrocautery Ground Pad - _____

G. 5-Lead ECG Electrodes - _____

3. Show the area that will be prepped by lightly shading it in on Tony's figure. Why is it important to consider the skin prep when placing monitors?

_____
_____
_____
_____

Skill Assessment 6-1

Sellick's Maneuver

Student Name _____ Date _____

Instructor _____

Procedural Step	Adequate	Needs Review
1. Student is able to define Sellick's Maneuver		
2. Verbalize purpose of Sellick's Maneuver		
3. Give two examples in which Sellick's Maneuver may be indicated		
4. Position self properly		
5. Identify relevant anatomy		
6. Position hand properly		
7. Apply adequate pressure		
8. Maintain cricoid pressure until asked to release		

Comments _____

_____

_____

_____

Skill Assessment 6-2

Draw Up Medication In A Syringe
(Off the Sterile Field)

Student Name _____ Date _____

Instructor _____

Procedural Step	Adequate	Needs Review
1. Student is able to provide pertinent information about the medication ordered		
2. Secure the ordered medication and all necessary supplies		
3. Verify that the "five rights" are met		
4. Verify that patient is not allergic to ordered medication		
5. Prepare medication container for withdrawal of medication		
6. Withdraw medication from container		
7. Needle for injection is applied to the syringe		
8. Medication label information is rechecked for accuracy		
9. Medication is labeled according to facility policy		

Comments _____
_____
_____
_____

Skill Assessment 6-3

Draw Up Medication In A Syringe
(Into the Sterile Field)

Student Name _____ Date _____

Instructor _____

Procedural Step	Adequate	Needs Review
1. Student is able to provide pertinent information about the medication ordered		
2. Secure the ordered medication and all necessary supplies		
3. Verify that the "five rights" are met		
4. Verify that patient is not allergic to ordered medication		
5. Circulator prepares medication container for withdrawal of medication		
6. STSR and circulator visually and verbally identify medication		
7. STSR withdraws medication from container		
8. STSR and circulator visually and verbally identify medication		
9. Needle for injection is applied to the syringe (if necessary)		
10. Medication is labeled according to facility policy		
11. Medication is passed to surgeon when requested and properly verbally identified		

Comments _____
_____
_____
_____

Skill Assessment 6-4

Accept Medication Into The Sterile Field
(Into a Container)

Student Name _____ Date _____

Instructor _____

Procedural Step	Adequate	Needs Review
1. Student is able to provide pertinent information about the medication ordered		
2. Secure the ordered medication and all necessary supplies		
3. Verify that the "five rights" are met		
4. Verify that patient is not allergic to ordered medication		
5. Circulator prepares medication for transfer to the sterile field		
6. STSR and circulator visually and verbally identify medication		
7. STSR presents container for acceptance of medication		
8. Medication is transferred to sterile field		
9. STSR and circulator visually and verbally identify medication		
10. Medication is correctly diluted (if necessary)		
11. Medication container is labeled according to facility policy		
12. Medication is prepared for use and additionally labeled (if necessary)		
13. Medication is passed to surgeon when requested and properly verbally identified		

Comments _____
_____
_____
_____

CHAPTER 7

Instrumentation, Equipment, and Supplies

OBJECTIVES

After studying this chapter, the reader should be able to:

C 1. Discuss the relationship between instrumentation, equipment, and supplies and quality patient care in the OR.

A 2. Identify items that require sterilization prior to use in the sterile field.

R 3. Identify basic instruments by type, function, and name.

4. Demonstrate proper care, handling, and assembly of instruments.

5. Identify types of special equipment utilized in OR practice and demonstrate proper care, handling techniques, and safety precautions.

6. Identify the names and functions of accessory equipment and demonstrate proper care, handling, and assembly.

7. Identify and prepare supplies used in the OR.

E 8. Discuss the relationship between instruments, equipment, and supplies and the OR environment as related to safety.

CHAPTER 7

■ Key Words

Define the following:

1. Ancillary _____
2. Aperture _____
3. Bipolar Cautery _____
4. Capillarity _____
5. Catheter _____
6. Cottonoid _____
7. Cryo- _____
8. Defibrillator _____
9. Drain _____
10. Fenestration _____
11. Insufflation _____
12. Irrigation _____
13. Magnification _____
14. Monopolar Cautery _____
15. Nd:YAG _____
16. Pneumatic _____
17. Resistance _____
18. Retract _____
19. Scalpel _____
20. Serrations (on a surgical instrument) _____
21. Stainless Steel _____
22. Teeth (on a surgical instrument) _____
23. Tube _____
24. Ureteral _____
25. Urethral _____

Exercise A – Identification

1. Identify the components of the instrument shown in Figure 7-1.

Figure 7-1

A. _____

B. _____

C. _____

D. _____

E. _____

2. Classify the instruments listed using the following designations:

Accessory   Clamping   Cutting   Dilating
   Grasping/Holding   Probing   Retracting
        Suctioning   Suturing

A. #3 Knife Handle _____

B. Allis _____

C. Babcock _____

D. Crile _____

E. Deaver _____

F. Debakey Tissue Forceps _____

G. Kocher _____

H. Metzenbaum _____

I. Mosquito _____

J. Needle Holder _____

K. Poole _____

L. Richardson _____

M. Towel Clamp _____

N. Yankauer _____

3. Organize the following instruments by size from shortest/smallest to longest/largest.

A. _____ Crile

B. _____ Mosquito

C. _____ Pean

D. _____ Schnidt

4. A #20 knife blade fits on a # _____ knife handle.

5. A #15 knife blade fits on a # _____ knife handle.

6. An oscillating saw uses a(n) _____ motion.

7. A reciprocating saw uses a(n) _____ motion.

8. The acronym "laser" represents _____ _____.

9. Trace the path of the electrical current when a unipolar electrosurgical unit is in use by placing the following elements in the correct order.

A. _____ Active Electrode

B. _____ Dispersive Electrode

C. _____ Generator

D. _____ Generator

E. _____ Ground

F. _____ Patient

70 CHAPTER 7

10. Identify the types of sponges shown in Figure 7-2.

    A. _____

    B. _____

Figure 7-2

■ Case Studies

☐ CASE STUDY 1

Edward has been assigned to prepare the Cysto Room for a transurethral resection of the prostate (TURP) using the Nd:YAG laser.

1. What does Nd:YAG represent?

   _____
   _____
   _____
   _____

2. What precautions must be taken to protect the patient and staff from the laser beam?

   _____
   _____
   _____
   _____

3. Will the laser be attached to the endoscope?

   _____
   _____
   _____
   _____

CASE STUDY 2

Madelena is preparing the OR for a neurosurgical procedure (carpal tunnel release). Both the unipolar and bipolar electrocautery units are requested on the surgeon's preference card.

1. Will Madelena need two grounding pads (dispersive electrodes)? Why or why not?

2. The patient will be placed in the supine position for the procedure. What anatomic site is the most likely place to affix the grounding pad(s)?

3. The surgeon's preference card requests that a tourniquet be available for the procedure. List at least three items that Madelena will need to facilitate the use of the tourniquet.

Skill Assessment 7-1

Assemble An Instrument Set

Student Name _____ Date _____

Instructor _____

Procedural Step	Adequate	Needs Review
1. Student is able to state purpose for assembling an instrument set in prescribed manner		
2. Appropriate attire		
3. Wash hands (Standard Precautions)		
4. Equipment and supplies assembled		
5. Organize workspace		
6. Assemble set		
7. Sign/initial count sheet/instrument list		
8. Place internal indicator		
9. Proceed with other tasks		

Comments _____

_____

_____

_____

Skill Assessment 7-2

Instrument Handling – Load, Pass, and Unload A Knife Handle

Student Name _____ Date _____

Instructor _____

Procedural Step	Adequate	Needs Review
1. Equipment and supplies assembled		
2. Student selects necessary items		
3. Knife blade is secured		
4. Blade is applied to knife handle		
5. Proceed with case preparation or case		
6. Scalpel is held in safe manner		
7. Scalpel is passed or placed for transfer		
8. Scalpel is retrieved		
9. Knife blade is removed from handle		
10. Discard knife blade		
11. Proceed with case or case breakdown		

Comments _____
_____
_____
_____

Skill Assessment 7-3

Instrument Handling – Recognize, Prepare, and Pass Various Types of Instruments (Sharps, Scissors, Tissue Forceps, Ringed Instruments, and Retractors)

Student Name _____ Date _____

Instructor _____

Procedural Step	Adequate	Needs Review
1. Equipment and supplies assembled		
2. Mayo stand is set up		
3. Student is able to recognize instruments by name		
4. Student secures instrument requested		
5. Pass sharp instruments or supplies		
6. Pass scissors		
7. Pass tissue forceps		
8. Pass ringed instrument(s)		
9. Pass retractor(s)		
10. Return items to storage location		
11. Attend to other intraoperative actions as needed		

Comments _____
_____
_____
_____

CHAPTER 8

Wound Healing, Sutures, Needles, and Stapling Devices

OBJECTIVES

After studying this chapter, the reader should be able to:

C 1. Define terms relevant to wound healing.

2. List the possible complications of wound healing.

A 3. Explain the classifications of surgical wounds.

4. Define and give examples of types of traumatic wounds.

5. List the factors that influence healing and describe the manner in which they affect the healing process.

R 6. Describe the characteristics of inflammation.

7. List and define common suture terms.

8. Identify suture materials and stapling devices and their usage.

9. Describe the types, characteristics, and uses of natural and synthetic absorbable suture materials.

10. List and describe the common natural and synthetic nonabsorbable sutures, stating their sources, common trade names, and uses.

11. Discuss preparation and handling techniques for suturing and stapling devices, and list the factors relating to the choice of each.

12. Identify, describe the use, and demonstrate proper handling of the various types of surgical needles.

13. List and define common suture techniques.

14. Discuss the basic uses and advantages of stapling instruments.

E 15. List the types of injury that cause damage to tissues.

16. List the characteristics of the types of healing.

17. Describe the stages/phases of wound healing.

CHAPTER 8

■ Key Terms

Define the following:

1. Adhesion _____
_____

2. Anastomosis _____
_____

3. Approximation _____
_____

4. Chromic _____
_____

5. Chronic Wound _____
_____

6. Cicatrix _____
_____

7. Dead Space _____
_____

8. Debridement _____
_____

9. Dehiscence _____
_____

10. Devitalized _____
_____

11. Evisceration _____
_____

12. First Intention _____
_____

13. Fray _____
_____

14. French Eye _____
_____

15. Friable _____
_____

16. Herniation _____
_____

17. Immunosuppressed Patient _____
_____

18. Inflammation _____
_____

19. Laceration _____
_____

20. Ligate _____
_____

21. Monofilament _____
_____

22. Packing _____
_____

23. Primary Suture Line _____
_____

24. PTFE _____
_____

25. Second Intention _____
_____

26. Secondary Suture Line _____
_____

27. Swaged _____
_____

28. Tensile Strength _____
_____

29. Third Intention _____
_____

30. Vessel Loop _____
_____

Case Studies

CASE STUDY 1

James, a 12-year-old male, lost control of his trail bike while riding on a course that he and some friends constructed in a vacant lot. He flew over the handlebars into the dirt onto his left arm. His arm is broken, and the bone is sticking out through the skin. It is 10:00 AM.

1. James has suffered a traumatic injury to his left arm. What classification(s) does his wound fall into?

   _____
   _____
   _____
   _____

2. James was immediately taken to the Urgent Care Center. It is determined that James will need surgical treatment and will be transferred by ambulance to the nearest hospital, which is 150 miles away. The surgery is scheduled for 4:00 PM. How will the surgical wound be classified? Why?

   _____
   _____
   _____
   _____

3. Is James at risk for surgical site infection? Why? What steps can be taken to minimize the risk of SSI?

   _____
   _____
   _____
   _____

CASE STUDY 2

Dorothea just had her ruptured appendix removed. The skin and subcutaneous layers of her wound have been left open. Her surgeon told her that if her wound showed no signs of infection in five days he would finish the closure.

1. Why did the surgeon leave the wound partially open? In its present condition, by what method is the wound expected to heal?

2. What signs will the surgeon use to determine if Dorothea's wound may be closed in five days?

3. If the wound can be closed in five days, what type of healing will then be expected? Is the tissue expected to regain normal tensile strength?

Skill Assessment 8-1

Suture/Needle/Staple Handling – Load, Pass, and Unload A Needle Holder

Student Name _____ Date _____

Instructor _____

Procedural Step	Adequate	Needs Review
1. Equipment and supplies assembled		
2. Select necessary items		
3. Open suture packet		
4. Needle holder is applied		
5. Suture is removed from packet		
6. Pass suture		
7. Companion instruments passed		
8. Suture is retrieved		
9. Needle holder is unloaded		
10. Return items to storage location		
11. Attend to other intraoperative actions as needed		

Comments _____

_____

_____

_____

Skill Assessment 8-2

Suture/Needle/Staple Handling – Load Empty Needle, Thread Suture, Pass, and Reload

Student Name _____ Date _____

Instructor _____

Procedural Step	Adequate	Needs Review
1. Equipment and supplies assembled		
2. Select necessary items		
3. Open suture packet		
4. Needle is placed in needle holder		
5. Needle holder is moved to left hand		
6. Suture is threaded		
7. Pass suture		
8. Companion instruments passed		
9. Needle is retrieved		
10. Reset needle and reload (if necessary)		
11. Needle holder is unloaded		
12. Return items to storage location		
13. Attend to other intraoperative actions as needed		

Comments _____

_____

_____

_____

Skill Assessment 8-3

Suture/Needle/Staple Handling – Pass Ties
(Includes Reel, Free Ties, and Ties on a Pass)

Student Name _____ Date _____

Instructor _____

Procedural Step	Adequate	Needs Review
1. Equipment and supplies assembled		
2. Select necessary items		
3. Prepare, pass, and retrieve reel		
4. Prepare and pass free tie		
5. Prepare and pass tie on a pass		
6. Attend to other intraoperative actions as needed		

Comments _____
_____
_____
_____

Skill Assessment 8-4

Suture/Needle/Staple Handling – Load, Pass, and Unload Various Types Of Stapling/Clipping Devices

Student Name _____ Date _____

Instructor _____

Procedural Step	Adequate	Needs Review
1. Equipment and supplies assembled		
2. Select necessary items		
3. Item is prepared for use		
4. Item is passed		
5. Item is retrieved		
6. Attend to other intraoperative actions as needed		

Comments _____

_____

_____

_____

CHAPTER 9

The Surgical Technologist in the Scrub Role (Case Management)

OBJECTIVES

After studying this chapter, the reader should be able to:

C 1. Describe the role of the STSR in caring for the surgical patient.

A 2. Demonstrate techniques of opening and preparing supplies and instruments needed for any operative procedure with the maintenance of sterile technique at all times.

3. Demonstrate the proper techniques for the surgical hand scrub, gowning, gloving, and assisting team members.

4. Demonstrate the proper technique for preparing supplies and instruments on a sterile field.

R 5. Demonstrate and explain in detail the procedure for counting instruments, sponges, needles, and other items on the sterile field.

6. Demonstrate the initial steps for starting a procedure.

7. Demonstrate intraoperative handling of sterile equipment and supplies.

E 8. Explain and demonstrate postoperative routines.

CHAPTER 9

■ Key Terms

Define the following:

1. Adhesive Drape _____

2. Anticipate _____

3. Antimicrobial _____

4. Biohazard _____

5. Circumferential _____

6. Craniotomy _____

7. Cylindrical _____

8. Don _____

9. Foreign Body _____

10. Handwash _____

11. Indicator _____

12. Lap Sponge _____

13. Mask _____

14. Neutral Zone _____

15. Pathology _____

16. PPE _____

17. Resident Organisms _____

18. Sterile Attire _____

19. Sterile Team Member _____

20. Stockinet _____

21. Surgeon Preference Card _____

22. Surgical Scrub _____

23. The Count _____

24. Transient Organisms _____

25. Wraparound-Style Gown _____

Case Studies

CASE STUDY 1

Sean is a student STSR for an LAVH. As he reaches for a supply item being handed by the circulator, his left glove touches the outside of the packet.

1. Does Sean have a problem? What is it?

2. What steps need to be taken to correct the problem?

3. Describe the procedure(s) for changing a contaminated glove.

CASE STUDY 2

It is LuAnn's big day. She is scrubbing her first case as a student. She wants desperately to do everything right.

1. What type of surgical scrub should LuAnn perform? Why?

2. Describe the counted brush stroke method for a surgical scrub.

3. Which method of self-gloving will LuAnn use after she has donned her sterile gown? Why?

Skill Assessment 9-1

Open Sterile Supplies – Back Table Pack

Student Name _____ Date _____

Instructor _____

Procedural Step	Adequate	Needs Review
1. Appropriate attire		
2. Wash hands (Standard Precautions)		
3. Equipment and supplies are assembled		
4. Check integrity of outer wrapper		
5. Remove dust cover		
6. Check integrity of inner package		
7. Orient pack on back table		
8. Open first fold and remove accessory items, if present		
9. Open second fold		
10. Open third fold		
11. Reposition self to open fourth fold		
12. Open fourth fold		
13. Proceed with case preparation		

Comments _____
_____
_____
_____

Skill Assessment 9-2

Open Sterile Supplies – Small Wrapped Package
(Such as Initial Gown – on Clean Surface)

Student Name _____ Date _____

Instructor _____

Procedural Step	Adequate	Needs Review
1. Appropriate attire		
2. Wash hands (Standard Precautions)		
3. Equipment and supplies assembled		
4. Check integrity of package		
5. Orient package on appropriate surface		
6. Open first fold		
7. Open second fold		
8. Open third fold		
9. Open fourth fold		
10. Proceed with case preparation		

Comments _____

_____

_____

_____

Skill Assessment 9-3

Open Sterile Supplies – Small Wrapped Package
(Onto Sterile Field or Secured by STSR)

Student Name _____ Date _____

Instructor _____

Procedural Step	Adequate	Needs Review
1. Appropriate attire		
2. Wash hands (Standard Precautions)		
3. Equipment and supplies assembled		
4. Check integrity of package		
5. Orient package properly in hand		
6. Open first fold, secure flap		
7. Open second fold, secure flap		
8. Open third fold, secure flap		
9. Open fourth fold, secure flap		
10. Approach sterile field/STSR		
11. Transfer item to sterile field/STSR		
12. Discard wrapper		
13. Proceed with case preparation		

Comments _____

_____

_____

_____

Skill Assessment 9-4

Open Sterile Supplies – Peel Pack

Student Name _____ Date _____

Instructor _____

Procedural Step	Adequate	Needs Review
1. Appropriate attire		
2. Wash hands (Standard Precautions)		
3. Equipment and supplies assembled		
4. Check integrity of package		
5. Orient package properly in both hands		
6. Slowly pull sides of peel pack away from each other		
7. Continue opening package		
8. Approach sterile field/STSR		
9. Transfer item to sterile field/STSR		
10. Discard wrapper		
11. Proceed with case preparation		

Comments _____

_____

_____

Skill Assessment 9-5

Open Sterile Supplies – Instrument Set (Container System)

Student Name _____ Date _____

Instructor _____

Procedural Step	Adequate	Needs Review
1. Appropriate attire		
2. Wash hands (Standard Precautions)		
3. Equipment and supplies assembled		
4. Check integrity of container		
5. Place instrument container on suitable surface		
6. Remove seals		
7. Release lid		
8. Lift lid		
9. Inspect interior of container		
10. Inspect lid		
11. Set lid in convenient location		
12. Proceed with case preparation		

Comments _____
_____
_____
_____

Skill Assessment 9-6

Open Sterile Supplies – Pour Sterile Solution

Student Name _____ Date _____

Instructor _____

Procedural Step	Adequate	Needs Review
1. Student is able to provide pertinent information about the sterile solution ordered		
2. Appropriate attire		
3. Wash hands (Standard Precautions)		
4. Equipment and supplies assembled		
5. Verify that the "five rights" are met		
6. Verify patient allergy status		
7. Remove protective outer seal from solution container		
8. Remove inner seal		
9. Approach sterile field		
10. STSR and circulator visually and verbally identify solution		
11. Pour sterile solution		
12. STSR and circulator visually and verbally identify solution		
13. Proceed with case preparation		

Comments _____

_____

_____

_____

Skill Assessment 9-7

Surgical Scrub – Counted Brush Stroke Method

Student Name _____ Date _____

Instructor _____

Procedural Step	Adequate	Needs Review
1. Student is able to define surgical scrub		
2. Student is able to state purpose for performing surgical scrub		
3. Appropriate attire		
4. Equipment and supplies are assembled		
5. Inspect integrity of hands and arms		
6. Open brush package		
7. Turn on water and adjust temperature		
8. Wet hands and arms, apply soap, lather		
9. Rinse		
10. Clean nails		
11. Secure and prepare brush		
12. Scrub nails of first hand		
13. Scrub fingers of first hand		
14. Scrub hand of first arm		
15. Scrub arm to 2" above elbow of first arm		
16. Transfer brush to scrubbed hand and scrub opposite extremity		
17. Discard brush		
18. Rinse		
19. Proceed to OR		

Comments _____

_____

_____

Skill Assessment 9-8

Gown – Self
(Dry, Don Gown and Gloves – Closed Glove Technique)

Student Name _____ Date _____

Instructor _____

Procedural Step	Adequate	Needs Review
1. Enter OR		
2. Secure towel		
3. Open towel		
4. Dry first hand and arm		
5. Transfer towel to opposite hand		
6. Dry opposite hand		
7. Discard towel		
8. Secure gown		
9. Unfold gown		
10. Don gown		
11. Secure first glove		
12. Position glove appropriately		
13. Don first glove		
14. Secure and don second glove		
15. Wrap around back of gown		
16. Proceed with case preparation		

Comments _____

_____

_____

Skill Assessment 9-9

Gown – Assist A Team Member
(Pass Towel, Apply Gown and Gloves – Open Glove Technique)

Student Name _____ Date _____

Instructor _____

Procedural Step	Adequate	Needs Review
1. Prepare items in advance of need		
2. Secure towel		
3. Open towel		
4. Present towel to team member		
5. Secure gown		
6. Unfold gown		
7. Present gown		
8. Secure right glove		
9. Prepare right glove		
10. Present right glove		
11. Secure, prepare, and present left glove		
12. Wrap around back of gown		
13. Remove lubricant (powder) from gloves		
14. Proceed with case preparation or case		

Comments _____

_____

_____

_____

Skill Assessment 9-10

Disrobe
(To Replace Sterile Attire During Case)

Student Name _____ Date _____

Instructor _____

Procedural Step	Adequate	Needs Review
1. Recognize that gloves and/or gown are contaminated during case		
2. Step away from sterile field and request new gown and appropriate size gloves		
3. Remain still, with back to circulator while gown is unfastened		
4. Face circulator; remain still while gown is removed		
5. Turn hands palm up and present one at a time to circulator (usually right hand first)		
6. Apply sterile gown and gloves		
7. Return to sterile field and continue with tasks		

Comments _____

_____

_____

_____

Skill Assessment 9-11

Disrobe
(End of Case)

Student Name _____ Date _____

Instructor _____

Procedural Step	Adequate	Needs Review
1. All tasks that require gown and gloves are complete		
2. Back of gown is unfastened		
3. Grasp gown near shoulders and roll away from self		
4. Remove gown (place gown in proper receptacle if feasible)		
5. Remove soiled gloves		
6. Grasp palm of glove to be removed first with opposite hand		
7. Remove first glove		
8. Keep removed glove in hand that remains gloved		
9. Begin to remove second glove		
10. Contain first glove inside of inverted second glove		
11. Finish removal of second glove		
12. Properly dispose of gown and gloves		
13. Wash hands (Standard Precautions)		

Comments _____
_____
_____
_____

The Surgical Technologist in the Scrub Role (Case Management) 117

Skill Assessment 9-12

Dress the Mayo Stand

Student Name _____ Date _____

Instructor _____

Procedural Step	Adequate	Needs Review
1. Equipment and supplies assembled		
2. Orient Mayo stand cover		
3. Insert hands in cuff of Mayo stand cover		
4. Secure folded edges of Mayo stand cover		
5. Approach Mayo stand		
6. Insert bare Mayo stand into prepared pocket of Mayo stand cover		
7. Slide Mayo stand cover onto Mayo stand		
8. Allow Mayo stand cover to unfold over back edge of stand		
9. Make final adjustments		
10. Place towels		
11. Proceed with case preparation		

Comments _____

_____

_____

_____

Skill Assessment 9-13

Fill A Bulb Syringe

Student Name _____ Date _____

Instructor _____

Procedural Step	Adequate	Needs Review
1. Equipment and supplies assembled		
2. Prepare bulb syringe		
3. Remove air		
4. Fill bulb syringe		
5. Proceed with case preparation or case		

Comments _____
_____
_____
_____

Skill Assessment 9-14

Remove Instrument Set From Container

Student Name _____ Date _____

Instructor _____

Procedural Step	Adequate	Needs Review
1. Equipment and supplies assembled		
2. Approach instrument container		
3. Secure instrument basket		
4. Step away from instrument container		
5. Place instrument basket on back table		
6. Proceed with case preparation or case		

Comments _____
_____
_____
_____

Skill Assessment 9-15

Case Management – Pre-Case Preparation
(Prior to Scrub)

Student Name _____ Date _____

Instructor _____

Procedural Step	Adequate	Needs Review
1. Appropriate attire		
2. Wash hands (Standard Precautions)		
3. Assignment received		
4. Secure surgeon preference card		
5. Locate case cart or assemble necessary items		
6. Verify that all items are present		
7. OR prepared for use		
8. Sterile items placed for use		
9. Open standard and specialty items		
10. Double-check supplies		
11. Proceed with case preparation		

Comments _____

_____

_____

_____

Skill Assessment 9-16

Case Management – Case Preparation
(Beginning with Surgical Scrub)

Student Name _____ Date _____

Instructor _____

Procedural Step	Adequate	Needs Review
1. Appropriate attire		
2. Sterility is maintained at all times		
3. Perform surgical scrub		
4. Proceed to OR		
5. Approach sterile field, secure towel, and dry self		
6. Don sterile gown		
7. Apply sterile gloves		
8. Prepare back table and basin set; dress Mayo stand		
9. Count necessary items		
10. Mayo stand prepared for use		
11. Preparation time less than 20 minutes		

Comments _____

_____

_____

_____

Skill Assessment 9-17

Case Management – Drape
(Basic Laparotomy)

Student Name _____ Date _____

Instructor _____

Procedural Step	Adequate	Needs Review
1. Equipment and supplies assembled		
2. Prepare drape materials		
3. Remains vigilant		
4. Report and correct problems immediately		
5. Hold drape materials at correct level		
6. Pass drape materials correctly		
7. Move safely between sterile fields		
8. Hand drapes in proper sequence		
9. Protect hands with drape cuff		
10. Communicate with team members as needed		
11. Other equipment is ready for placement		
12. Move furniture into position		
13. Proceed with case preparation or case		

Comments _____
_____
_____
_____

Skill Assessment 9-18

Case Management – Intraoperative Actions

Student Name _____ Date _____

Instructor _____

Procedural Step	Adequate	Needs Review
1. Equipment and supplies assembled		
2. Assist other team members to enter sterile field		
3. Perform tasks related to draping		
4. Place additional equipment on field as needed		
5. Move furniture into position		
6. Prepare field		
7. Pass scalpel		
8. Handle electrocautery properly		
9. Hand instruments correctly		
10. Prepare, identify, and handle all solutions correctly		
11. Prepare, identify, and handle all medications correctly		
12. Remove small sponges (if necessary)		
13. Respond to team member needs appropriately		
14. Communicate effectively with circulator		
15. Prepare, identify, and handle sutures and needles correctly		
16. Perform closing count(s)		
17. Report and correct problems immediately		
18. Maintain an orderly field		
19. Prepare for end of case		
20. Maintain sterile field until patient removed from OR		
21. Proceed with post-procedure actions		

Comments _____

_____

_____

_____

Skill Assessment 9-19

Case Management – Post-Procedure Actions

Student Name _____ Date _____

Instructor _____

Procedural Step	Adequate	Needs Review
1. Maintain sterile field until patient removed from OR		
2. Remove drapes from patient		
3. Assist with patient care as needed		
4. Return to tasks related to breakdown of field		
5. Handle all materials safely		
6. All sharps disposed of correctly		
7. Handle all biohazardous waste (linen and trash) correctly		
8. Follow policy for instrument care		
9. Remove gown and gloves properly		
10. Wash hands (Standard Precautions)		
11. Care for equipment as needed		
12. Follow OR cleaning/turn-over procedure		

Comments _____

_____

_____

_____

CHAPTER 10

Diagnostic Procedures

OBJECTIVES

After studying this chapter, the reader should be able to:

A 1. Apply knowledge of anatomy and physiology to determine which diagnostic examinations will be useful.

P 2. List the sources of patient data.

3. List and discuss techniques used to establish the diagnosis.

O 4. Determine which diagnostic procedures will require surgical intervention.

5. Identify the major indications for surgical intervention.

S 6. Understand the surgical technologist's role in caring for each specific type of specimen.

Key Terms

Define the following:

1. Angina _____
2. Auscultation _____
3. Biopsy _____
4. Capnography _____
5. C-Arm _____
6. Cholangiography _____
7. Contrast Media _____
8. CSF _____
9. Cystoscopy _____
10. ECG _____
11. EEG _____
12. Frozen Section _____
13. -gram _____
14. Gram's Stain _____
15. -graph _____
16. Indwelling _____
17. Isotope Scanning _____
18. Obstruction _____
19. Palpation _____
20. Prosthesis _____
21. Roentgenography _____
22. Sign _____
23. Symptom _____
24. UA _____
25. Ultrasonography _____

Diagnostic Procedures 135

Exercise A – Anatomy

1. Identify the structures of the biliary tract shown in Figure 10-1.

Figure 10-1

A. _____   B. _____

C. _____   D. _____

E. _____   F. _____

2. What type of radiographic exam would be used to visualize the structures of the biliary tract?

_____

_____

3. Identify the bony structures shown in Figure 10-2.

A. _____   B. _____

C. _____   D. _____

E. _____   F. _____

4. What radiographic view is shown in Figure 10-2, and which structure(s) is/are the primary focus of the exam? _____

_____

_____

Figure 10-2

5. Identify the bony structures shown in Figure 10-3.

Figure 10-3

A. _____   B. _____

C. _____   D. _____

E. _____   F. _____

6. What radiographic view is shown in Figure 10-3?

_____

_____

136   **CHAPTER 10**

7. In what position was the patient placed in order to obtain the radiographic view shown in Figure 10-3? _____

8. Identify the structures of the urinary system shown in Figure 10-4.

Figure 10-4

    A. _____   B. _____

    C. _____   D. _____

    E. _____   F. _____

9. Has contrast been used to obtain the radiograph shown in Figure 10-4? _____

10. In what position was the patient placed in order to obtain the radiographic view shown in Figure 10-4? _____

11. Figure 10-5 shows an image of the liver. How was this image obtained? _____

Figure 10-5

12. Why is ultrasonography ideal for examination of the fetus? _____

13. What piece of radiographic equipment is shown in Figure 10-6? _____

14. What is the advantage of fluoroscopy? _____

Figure 10-6

15. Locate the following structures in the correct abdominal quadrant.

    RUQ = Right Upper Quadrant
    LUQ = Left Upper Quadrant
    RLQ = Right Lower Quadrant
    LLQ = Left Lower Quadrant

    A. Gallbladder _____   B. Spleen _____

    C. Appendix _____   D. Liver _____

    E. Stomach _____   F. Left Ovary _____

■ Exercise B – Pathology

1. What pathologic condition(s) is/are detected with the use of cholecystography? _____

2. What type of examination is necessary to identify a pneumothorax? _____

3. What type of examination(s) would a patient experiencing a possible ureteral obstruction undergo to confirm the diagnosis? _____

4. What is the one condition that an MIBG scan is useful in diagnosing? _____

5. Will pressure readings from a Swan-Ganz catheter placed in the pulmonary artery be useful in diagnosing pulmonary embolism? _____

6. What is the purpose of performing a Gram's stain? _____

7. The patient is suspected to have a spinal cord tumor. Will an MRI or a CT scan be more useful in visualizing the soft tissue tumor? _____

8. What is considered the first step in determining the etiology of a patient's condition? Why? _____

9. Three types of visualization may be used by the examiner during a physical exam. Name the three types, explain how they differ, list any special equipment that may be needed for each, and give at least one example of each type.

    A. _____

    B. _____

    C. _____

10. To confirm a preliminary diagnosis of deep vein thrombosis, what diagnostic examination will be ordered by the physician? _____

11. A bone scan is an example of what type of scan? The term "hot spot" refers to what aspect of the scan, and what condition might be indicated by its presence? _____

12. Name the two methods of administering radiation therapy. What is the purpose of administering radiation therapy? _____

138 CHAPTER 10

13. The physician has ordered a blood gas study. Will the blood be drawn from a venous or arterial source? _____

14. What is the normal amount of glucose expected in a urine sample? Use Table 10–3 from the textbook to determine your answer. _____

15. A "culture and sensitivity" has been ordered. The organism has been "cultured" and identified. What is determined by the "sensitivity" portion of the exam? _____

■ Exercise C – Operation

1. Name the five types of cholecystography.

   A. _____ B. _____

   C. _____ D. _____

   E. _____

2. What purpose does a "scout" film (X-ray) serve? _____

3. Is transesophageal echocardiography an invasive procedure? Why? _____

4. What does the term "noninvasive" mean? _____

5. What is the ideal location for insertion of a Swan-Ganz pulmonary artery catheter? List two alternative locations. _____

6. List four intraoperative applications for fluoroscopy.

   A. _____

   B. _____

   C. _____

   D. _____

7. Explain the difference(s) between incisional biopsy and excisional biopsy. _____

8. The surgeon has requested that fluid aspirated from the thoracic cavity be sent to the laboratory to be cultured for aerobic and anaerobic organisms. What special supplies (if any) will be needed? _____

9. The surgeon has requested a frozen section on a piece of breast tissue that has been excised. Will the specimen be placed in formalin? Why? _____

10. Why is it necessary for the pathologist to be readily available to perform a frozen section? _____

11. A six-month-old is scheduled to undergo a CT scan with general anesthesia. What is the most likely reason that general anesthesia will be administered? _____

12. Explain the difference between a diagnostic and therapeutic procedure. _____

13. List the steps, in order, for percutaneous placement of a femoral artery catheter using the Seldinger technique.

   A. _____

   B. _____

   C. _____

   D. _____

   E. _____

   F. _____

   G. _____

   H. _____

14. What is the difference between a simple voided urine specimen and a clean-catch specimen? What supplies are needed for each? _____

   _____

   _____

   _____

15. Panendoscopy of the upper aerodigestive tract has been scheduled. What structures will be visualized, and what, if any, specialized equipment will be needed? _____

   _____

   _____

140   CHAPTER 10

■ Exercise D – Specific Variations

Student Name _____ Date _____

Instructor _____

Surgical Procedure – Student Case Study Report

The student will be provided with basic patient information (real or simulated) and is expected to complete the following case study.

1. Procedure name: _____
   _____
   _____

2. Definition of procedure: _____
   _____
   _____
   _____

3. What is the purpose of the procedure? _____
   _____
   _____
   _____

4. What is the expected outcome of the procedure?
   _____
   _____
   _____
   _____

5. Patient age: _____

6. Gender: _____

7. Additional pertinent patient information: ____
   _____
   _____
   _____

8. Probable preoperative diagnosis: _____
   _____
   _____
   _____
   _____
   _____

9. How was the diagnosis determined? _____
   _____
   _____
   _____
   _____
   _____

10. Discuss the relevant anatomy. _____
    _____
    _____
    _____
    _____
    _____
    _____

11. List the general and procedure-specific equipment that will be needed for the procedure.

    _____   _____
    _____   _____
    _____   _____
    _____   _____
    _____   _____

12. List the general and procedure-specific instruments that will be needed for the procedure.

    _____ _____
    _____ _____
    _____ _____
    _____ _____
    _____ _____
    _____

13. List the basic and procedure-specific supplies that will be needed for the procedure.

    Pack _____

    Basin _____

    Gloves _____

    Blades _____

    Drapes _____

    _____

    Drains _____

    Dressings _____

    _____

    Suture – Type of Suture, Needle (if applicable), and Anticipated Tissue Usage

    _____ _____
    _____ _____
    _____ _____
    _____ _____
    _____ _____
    _____ _____

    Pharmaceuticals

    _____ _____
    _____ _____
    _____ _____
    _____ _____

    Miscellaneous

    _____ _____
    _____ _____
    _____ _____
    _____ _____
    _____ _____
    _____

14. Operative preparation: _____
    _____
    _____
    _____
    _____
    _____
    _____
    _____

15. What type of anesthesia will likely be used? Why?
    _____
    _____
    _____
    _____
    _____
    _____

16. List any special anesthesia equipment that may be needed. _____
    _____
    _____
    _____
    _____
    _____
    _____

17. Patient position during the procedure: _____
    _____
    _____
    _____

142 CHAPTER 10

18. What supplies will be necessary for positioning?
_____
_____
_____
_____
_____

19. What type of shave/skin preparation will be necessary (if any)? _____
_____
_____
_____
_____
_____

20. Define the anatomic perimeters of the prep.
_____
_____
_____
_____
_____

21. List the order in which the drapes will be applied, and describe any specific variations.
_____
_____
_____
_____
_____
_____
_____

22. List any practical considerations.
_____
_____
_____
_____
_____
_____
_____

23. List the procedural steps, and describe the preparatory and supportive actions of the STSR during each step (use additional space if necessary).

Operative Procedure	Technical Considerations
1.	•
	•
2.	•
	•
3.	•
	•
4.	•
	•
5.	•
	•

Operative Procedure *continued*	**Technical Considerations** *continued*
6.	•
	•
7.	•
	•
8.	•
	•
9.	•
	•
10.	•
	•

24. What is the postoperative diagnosis? _____

_____

_____

_____

_____

25. Describe the immediate postoperative care.

_____

_____

_____

_____

26. What is the patient's long-term prognosis?

_____

_____

_____

_____

27. What are the possible complications? _____

_____

_____

_____

_____

28. Comments or questions: _____

_____

_____

_____

_____

29. What is the most valuable information you obtained from preparing this surgical procedure case study? _____

_____

_____

_____

144　CHAPTER 10

Case Studies

☐ CASE STUDY 1

Paul, a young athlete, has been scheduled for surgical removal of a Baker's cyst.

1. What is a Baker's cyst?

2. What diagnostic radiographic exam may have been performed to diagnose Paul's cyst?

3. In what position will Paul be placed to remove the Baker's cyst?

CASE STUDY 2

Lynn has just suffered a fall off a stepladder. She fell backwards, striking her head against the wall. She temporarily lost consciousness but is now awake, alert, and oriented. Lynn was transferred to the emergency department at the local hospital by ambulance with a cervical collar in place. She responds appropriately to verbal commands and is able to move all four extremities.

1. Lynn is complaining that the collar is too tight. Should it be removed? Why?

2. What diagnostic examination must be performed prior to removal of the cervical collar?

3. What type of physician specialist will be needed to interpret the results of the diagnostic exam?

General Surgery

CHAPTER 11

OBJECTIVES

After studying this chapter, the reader should be able to:

A 1. Discuss the relevant anatomy and physiology of the abdominal wall, digestive system, hepatic and biliary system, pancreas, spleen, thyroid and breast.

P 2. Describe the pathology and related terminology of each system or organ that prompts surgical intervention.

3. Discuss any preoperative diagnostic procedures and tests.

4. Discuss any special preoperative preparation procedures related to general surgery procedure.

O 5. Identify the names and uses of general surgery instruments, supplies, and drugs.

6. Identify the names and uses of special equipment related to general surgery.

7. Discuss the intraoperative preparation of the patient undergoing general surgical procedure.

8. Define and give an overview of illustrative general surgery procedures.

9. Discuss the purpose and expected outcomes of the illustrative procedures.

10. Discuss the immediate postoperative care and possible complications of the illustrative procedures.

S 11. Discuss any specific variations related to the preoperative, intraoperative, and postoperative care of the general surgery patient.

Key Terms

Define the following:

1. Absorption _____
2. Anastomosis _____
3. Ascites _____
4. Bile _____
5. Chole- _____
6. Chyle _____
7. Chyme _____
8. -cysto _____
9. -docho _____
10. -ectomy _____
11. Excision _____
12. Incision _____

13. Lysis _____
14. Necrosis _____
15. -oma _____
16. -ostomy _____
17. -otomy _____
18. Parietal _____
19. Peristalsis _____
20. Peritoneum _____
21. Portal System _____
22. Stasis _____
23. Stenosis _____
24. Ulcer _____
25. Viscera _____

Exercise A – Anatomy

1. Trace the alimentary pathway by placing the following elements in the correct order.

   A. _____ Anus
   B. _____ Ascending colon
   C. _____ Body of stomach
   D. _____ Cardia of stomach
   E. _____ Cardiac sphincter
   F. _____ Cecum
   G. _____ Descending colon
   H. _____ Duodenum
   I. _____ Epiglottis
   J. _____ Esophagus
   K. _____ Fundus of stomach
   L. _____ Hepatic flexure
   M. _____ Ileocecal valve
   N. _____ Ileum
   O. _____ Jejunum
   P. _____ Labia
   Q. _____ Mouth
   R. _____ Pharynx
   S. _____ Pyloric sphincter
   T. _____ Pylorus of stomach
   U. _____ Rectum
   V. _____ Sigmoid colon
   W. _____ Splenic flexure
   X. _____ Transverse colon
   Y. _____ Uvula

2. Identify the accessory digestive ducts and organs shown in Figure 11-1.

   A. _____   B. _____
   C. _____   D. _____
   E. _____   F. _____
   G. _____   H. _____
   I. _____   J. _____

Figure 11-1

150 CHAPTER 11

Figure 11-2 Thyroid Gland

Figure 11-3 Intestinal Wall

3. Identify the structures shown in Figure 11-2.

   A. _____   B. _____
   C. _____   D. _____
   E. _____   F. _____
   G. _____   H. _____
   I. _____   J. _____
   K. _____   L. _____
   M. _____   N. _____

4. Identify the components of the intestinal wall shown in Figure 11-3.

   A. _____   B. _____
   C. _____   D. _____
   E. _____   F. _____
   G. _____   H. _____
   I. _____   J. _____
   K. _____

5. The gallbladder is located in the _____ _____ quadrant of the abdomen.

6. Linea alba literally means _____ _____ and will be found in the _____ abdominal wall.

7. Parasympathetic innervation to the stomach is provided by the _____ nerve.

8. The four layers of the wall of the colon are _____, _____, _____, and _____.

9. The pancreas is classified as both a(n) _____ and _____ gland.

10. What is the primary function of the peritoneum?
    _____
    _____

11. Name the five sections of the stomach.

    A. _____
    B. _____
    C. _____
    D. _____
    E. _____

12. Where are the islets of Langerhans located, and what is their function? _____

13. What is the largest organ in the normal abdominal cavity? _____

14. List the functions that are performed by the cells of the liver.

    A. _____
    B. _____
    C. _____
    D. _____
    E. _____
    F. _____

15. What is the function of the sphincter of Oddi? _____

■ Exercise B – Pathology

1. Peptic ulcers are most frequently found in which location? _____

2. Explain the difference between an incarcerated and a strangulated hernia. _____

3. Is a direct hernia congenital or acquired? _____

4. What is diverticulitis? _____

5. What causes intra-abdominal adhesions? _____

6. Are a hemorrhoid and a pile the same? _____

7. What are the two types of choleliths, and what is the composition of each?

    A. _____
    B. _____

8. What is "referred" pain? _____

9. What is the usual cause of appendicitis? _____

10. Thrombocytopenia is a deficiency of _____ in the blood.

11. Which diagnostic tools will be useful in determining liver pathology? _____

12. List four of the causes of varicose veins of the lower extremity.

    A. _____
    B. _____
    C. _____
    D. _____

13. Define gynecomastia, and describe the surgical treatment that may be recommended to treat the condition. _____

14. Overactivity of the thyroid gland is referred to as _____

152   CHAPTER 11

15. What is meant by the term "staging" in reference to malignant tumors? _____

■ Exercise C – Operation

1. Laparoscopic Nissen fundoplication is performed to treat which condition(s)? _____

2. What structure is dilated with a Maloney dilator? Is the Maloney dilator inserted under sterile conditions? Why? _____

3. List two reasons for performing a gastrostomy.

   A. _____

   B. _____

4. Explain what is meant by the phrase "mobilize the bowel." _____

5. List the three basic configurations for intestinal anastomosis.

   A. _____

   B. _____

   C. _____

6. Describe the technique used to care for instrumentation and supplies that have been exposed to the inside of the intestinal tract. _____

7. What is a stoma? _____

8. What is the purpose of a T-tube, and where is it placed? _____

9. Why is it important to expel all air from the cholangiogram system prior to an intraoperative cholangiogram? _____

10. What is the reason for providing a second setup to perform a breast reconstruction following a modified radical mastectomy due to a malignancy? _____

11. Why is it important for the STSR to maintain the sterile field until the patient is extubated and breathing freely following a thyroidectomy? _____

12. What instruments and supplies will be needed to enter the common bile duct for CBDE? _____

13. Name the two positions that provide access to the anus.

    A. _____

    B. _____

14. What type of procedure is performed through a McBurney's incision? _____

15. McVay repair is performed to correct which condition? _____

Exercise D – Specific Variations

Student Name _____ Date _____

Instructor _____

Surgical Procedure – Student Case Study Report

The student will be provided with basic patient information (real or simulated) and is expected to complete the following case study.

1. Procedure name: _____
   _____
   _____

2. Definition of procedure: _____
   _____
   _____
   _____

3. What is the purpose of the procedure? _____
   _____
   _____
   _____

4. What is the expected outcome of the procedure?
   _____
   _____
   _____

5. Patient age: _____

6. Gender: _____

7. Additional pertinent patient information: _____
   _____
   _____

8. Probable preoperative diagnosis: _____
   _____
   _____
   _____
   _____
   _____

9. How was the diagnosis determined? _____
   _____
   _____
   _____
   _____

10. Discuss the relevant anatomy. _____
    _____
    _____
    _____
    _____

11. List the general and procedure-specific equipment that will be needed for the procedure.

    _____ _____
    _____ _____
    _____ _____
    _____ _____
    _____ _____

154 CHAPTER 11

12. List the general and procedure-specific instruments that will be needed for the procedure.

   _____   _____
   _____   _____
   _____   _____
   _____   _____
   _____   _____
   _____

13. List the basic and procedure-specific supplies that will be needed for the procedure.

   Pack _____
   Basin _____
   Gloves _____
   Blades _____
   Drapes _____
   _____
   Drains _____
   Dressings _____
   _____

   Suture – Type of Suture, Needle (if applicable), and Anticipated Tissue Usage

   _____   _____
   _____   _____
   _____   _____
   _____   _____
   _____   _____

   Pharmaceuticals

   _____   _____
   _____   _____
   _____   _____
   _____   _____

Miscellaneous

   _____   _____
   _____   _____
   _____   _____
   _____   _____
   _____   _____
   _____   _____

14. Operative preparation: _____
   _____
   _____
   _____
   _____
   _____
   _____
   _____

15. What type of anesthesia will likely be used? Why?
   _____
   _____
   _____
   _____
   _____

16. List any special anesthesia equipment that may be needed. _____
   _____
   _____
   _____
   _____
   _____
   _____

17. Patient position during the procedure: _____
   _____
   _____
   _____
   _____

18. What supplies will be necessary for positioning?
    _____
    _____
    _____
    _____

19. What type of shave/skin preparation will be necessary (if any)? _____
    _____
    _____
    _____
    _____

20. Define the anatomic perimeters of the prep.
    _____
    _____
    _____
    _____

21. List the order in which the drapes will be applied, and describe any specific variations.
    _____
    _____
    _____
    _____
    _____
    _____
    _____

22. List any practical considerations.
    _____
    _____
    _____
    _____
    _____
    _____

23. List the procedural steps, and describe the preparatory and supportive actions of the STSR during each step (use additional space if necessary).

Operative Procedure	Technical Considerations
1.	•
	•
2.	•
	•
3.	•
	•
4.	•
	•
5.	•
	•

Operative Procedure continued	**Technical Considerations** continued
6.	•
	•
7.	•
	•
8.	•
	•
9.	•
	•
10.	•
	•

24. What is the postoperative diagnosis? _____
_____
_____
_____
_____
_____

25. Describe the immediate postoperative care.
_____
_____
_____
_____
_____
_____

26. What is the patient's long-term prognosis?
_____
_____
_____
_____
_____

27. What are the possible complications? _____
_____
_____
_____
_____
_____
_____

28. Comments or questions: _____
_____
_____
_____
_____

29. What is the most valuable information you obtained from preparing this surgical procedure case study? _____
_____
_____
_____
_____

Case Studies

☐ CASE STUDY 1

Lin Su is a 21-year-old female college student. She was admitted to the college's health center for right lower quadrant pain, nausea, and low-grade fever. She was diagnosed with acute appendicitis, and surgery was scheduled.

1. What causes appendicitis?

2. What are the signs and symptoms of appendicitis?

3. Describe a McBurney's incision.

4. What is the primary difference between a McBurney's and a Rockey-Davis incision?

CHAPTER 11

CASE STUDY 2

Jon and Linda are both computer programmers and 41 years of age. They are in the preoperative holding area. Each is scheduled for a hernia repair in the groin area.

1. What are the chances that Jon's hernia is a femoral hernia?

2. Jon's hernia is said to be incarcerated. What does this mean?

3. If Linda has a femoral hernia, the hernia exists below what anatomic marker?

4. What is Hesselbach's triangle?

5. Jon's hernia was described in the postoperative report as a direct hernia. Is it probable that the hernia was congenital in nature?

CHAPTER 12

Obstetric and Gynecologic Surgery

OBJECTIVES

After studying this chapter, the reader should be able to:

A 1. Discuss the relevant anatomy and physiology of the female reproductive system.

P 2. Describe the pathology of the female reproductive system that prompts surgical intervention and the related terminology.

3. Discuss any special preoperative obstetric and gynecologic diagnostic procedures/tests.

O 4. Discuss any special preoperative preparation procedures related to obstetric/gynecologic procedures.

5. Identify the names and uses of obstetric and gynecologic instruments, supplies, and drugs.

6. Identify the names and uses of special equipment related to obstetric/gynecologic surgery.

7. Discuss the intraoperative preparation of the patient undergoing an obstetric or gynecologic procedure.

8. Define and give an overview of the obstetric/gynecologic procedure.

9. Discuss the purpose and expected outcomes of the obstetric/gynecologic procedure.

10. Discuss the immediate postoperative care and possible complications of the obstetric/gynecologic procedure.

S 11. Discuss any specific variations related to the preoperative, intraoperative, and postoperative care of the obstetric/gynecologic patient.

Key Terms

Define the following:

1. Adnexa _____
2. Bony Pelvis _____
3. Breech _____
4. Corpus Luteum _____
5. CPD _____
6. C-Section _____
7. Curettage _____
8. Delivery Forceps _____
9. DUB _____
10. Dystocia _____
11. Episiotomy _____
12. Exenteration _____
13. Fimbria _____
14. Fistula _____
15. Gravida _____
16. Human Chorionic Gonadotropin ___
17. LEEP _____
18. Ligament _____
19. Marsupialization _____
20. Myoma _____
21. Occiput Anterior _____
22. Parity _____
23. Perineum _____
24. Pfannenstiel _____
25. Vestibule _____

Exercise A – Anatomy

1. Identify the structures of the external female genitalia shown in Figure 12-1.

Figure 12-1

A. _____
B. _____
C. _____
D. _____
E. _____
F. _____
G. _____
H. _____
I. _____

2. Identify the structures shown in Figure 12-2.

A. _____
B. _____
C. _____
D. _____
E. _____
F. _____
G. _____

Figure 12-2

H. _____
I. _____
J. _____
K. _____
L. _____
M. _____
N. _____
O. _____
P. _____

3. Identify the structures of the female reproductive system shown in Figure 12-3.

Figure 12-3

CHAPTER 12

A. _____
B. _____
C. _____
D. _____
E. _____
F. _____
G. _____
H. _____
I. _____
J. _____
K. _____
L. _____
M. _____
N. _____
O. _____
P. _____
Q. _____
R. _____
S. _____

4. What is the fornix? _____
_____
_____

5. Describe the locations of the internal and external cervical os. _____
_____
_____

6. List the three layers of the uterine wall.

   A. _____
   B. _____
   C. _____

7. Where are the Bartholin's glands located? What is their function? _____
_____
_____

8. List the structures contained within the broad ligament.

   A. _____
   B. _____
   C. _____
   D. _____
   E. _____
   F. _____

9. What are the other two names for the fallopian tubes? _____
_____
_____

10. Describe the location of the ovaries. _____
_____
_____

11. Name the two hormones from the anterior pituitary that stimulate the ovarian cycle. _____
_____
_____

12. Name the two hormones that are produced by the ovary. _____
_____
_____

13. Name the bones of the pelvic girdle. _____
_____
_____

14. What is the main muscle of the pelvic floor? Name its three components. _____
_____

   A. _____
   B. _____
   C. _____

15. Branches of which nerve provide sensation to the perineum? _____
_____

Exercise B – Pathology

1. Are Braxton Hicks contractions an indication that delivery of the fetus is imminent? _____

2. Cord blood is collected routinely with every delivery. Why? _____

3. What does "fetal distress" mean? _____

4. What is the most common reason for performing a cesarean section? _____

5. Define "cystocele," and give two reasons why a cystocele may occur. _____

6. What condition is diagnosed with the use of the Pap smear? _____

7. List the possible sites for ectopic pregnancy. _____

8. What is meant by the term "incompetent cervix"? What procedure is performed to treat the condition during pregnancy? _____

9. Define "leiomyoma." _____

10. What are the symptoms of endometriosis? _____

11. Is ultrasound useful in diagnosing a malignancy? _____

12. What is the most common symptom of uterine cancer? _____

13. List two placental conditions that may necessitate a cesarean section. _____

14. Amenorrhea is the condition of _____.

15. What is a pedunculated lesion? _____

Exercise C – Operation

1. In what position will the patient be placed to accomplish a D&C? In addition to the basic position, which position may be used to enhance the surgeon's view of the anatomy? _____

2. Explain the usefulness of the Trendelenburg position during pelvic surgery. _____

3. Describe the complications that the patient may suffer from an undiagnosed or improperly-closed perineal laceration. _____

164   CHAPTER 12

4. Name two types of suction devices that may be used to clear a neonates' airway. _____

5. What are the advantages to a "classic" approach for a cesarean section? _____

6. Name the three approaches that are available for tubal sterilization.

   A. _____

   B. _____

   C. _____

7. Posterior colporrhaphy is performed to treat which condition? _____

8. What is Lugol's solution used for? _____

9. What are some advantages to LAVH? _____

10. What is the importance of draining the bladder prior to D&C? _____

11. Why is a Foley catheter placed prior to a cesarean section? _____

12. List the structures that will be removed during total pelvic exenteration. _____

13. What safety measures must be implemented when a laser is in use? _____

14. List the drape components that are necessary to drape a patient in the lithotomy position. Describe the draping sequence. _____

15. What structure(s) is/are removed during a TAH? _____

Exercise D – Specific Variations

Student Name _____ Date _____

Instructor _____

Surgical Procedure – Student Case Study Report

The student will be provided with basic patient information (real or simulated) and is expected to complete the following case study.

1. Procedure name: _____
   _____
   _____

2. Definition of procedure: _____
   _____
   _____
   _____

3. What is the purpose of the procedure? ____
   _____
   _____
   _____
   _____

4. What is the expected outcome of the procedure?
   _____
   _____
   _____
   _____

5. Patient age: _____

6. Gender: _____

7. Additional pertinent patient information: ___
   _____
   _____
   _____

8. Probable preoperative diagnosis: _____
   _____
   _____
   _____
   _____
   _____

9. How was the diagnosis determined? _____
   _____
   _____
   _____
   _____
   _____

10. Discuss the relevant anatomy. _____
    _____
    _____
    _____
    _____
    _____

11. List the general and procedure-specific equipment that will be needed for the procedure.

    _____   _____
    _____   _____
    _____   _____
    _____   _____
    _____   _____

166 CHAPTER 12

12. List the general and procedure-specific instruments that will be needed for the procedure.

   _____ _____
   _____ _____
   _____ _____
   _____ _____
   _____ _____
   _____

13. List the basic and procedure-specific supplies that will be needed for the procedure.

   Pack _____
   Basin _____
   Gloves _____
   Blades _____
   Drapes _____
   _____
   Drains _____
   Dressings _____
   _____

   Suture – Type of Suture, Needle (if applicable), and Anticipated Tissue Usage

   _____ _____
   _____ _____
   _____ _____
   _____ _____
   _____ _____
   _____ _____
   _____

   Pharmaceuticals

   _____ _____
   _____ _____
   _____ _____
   _____ _____

Miscellaneous

   _____ _____
   _____ _____
   _____ _____
   _____ _____
   _____ _____
   _____

14. Operative preparation: _____
   _____
   _____
   _____
   _____
   _____
   _____
   _____

15. What type of anesthesia will likely be used? Why?
   _____
   _____
   _____
   _____
   _____
   _____

16. List any special anesthesia equipment that may be needed. _____
   _____
   _____
   _____
   _____
   _____
   _____
   _____

17. Patient position during the procedure: _____
   _____
   _____
   _____
   _____

18. What supplies will be necessary for positioning?
    _____
    _____
    _____
    _____
    _____

19. What type of shave/skin preparation will be necessary (if any)? _____
    _____
    _____
    _____
    _____
    _____

20. Define the anatomic perimeters of the prep.
    _____
    _____
    _____
    _____
    _____
    _____

21. List the order in which the drapes will be applied, and describe any specific variations.
    _____
    _____
    _____
    _____
    _____
    _____
    _____
    _____

22. List any practical considerations.
    _____
    _____
    _____
    _____
    _____
    _____

23. List the procedural steps, and describe the preparatory and supportive actions of the STSR during each step (use additional space if necessary).

Operative Procedure	Technical Considerations
1.	•
	•
2.	•
	•
3.	•
	•
4.	•
	•
5.	•
	•

CHAPTER 12

Operative Procedure *continued*	Technical Considerations *continued*
6.	•
	•
7.	•
	•
8.	•
	•
9.	•
	•
10.	•
	•

24. What is the postoperative diagnosis? _____

25. Describe the immediate postoperative care.

26. What is the patient's long-term prognosis?

27. What are the possible complications? _____

28. Comments or questions: _____

29. What is the most valuable information you obtained from preparing this surgical procedure case study? _____

Case Studies

CASE STUDY 1

Shannon is a 23-year-old primipara who has just been admitted to the labor and delivery unit. She has had a normal pregnancy, and sonograms confirm only one fetus. Her cervix is dilated to 4 cm.

1. How long, on average, would you expect her labor to continue?

2. To what does the term "presentation" refer?

3. To what does the term "position" refer?

4. To what does the term "station" refer?

CHAPTER 12

☐ CASE STUDY 2

Correta has been admitted for a diagnostic laparoscopy for pelvic pain of unknown origin.

1. What equipment will be needed for the procedure?

2. What instruments will be needed for the procedure?

3. In what position will the Correta be placed?

4. What are the common complications of laparoscopy?

Ophthalmic Surgery

CHAPTER 13

OBJECTIVES

After studying this chapter, the reader should be able to:

A 1. Discuss the anatomy of the eye.

P 2. Describe the pathology that prompts surgical intervention of the eye and related terminology.

3. Discuss any special preoperative ophthalmic diagnostic procedures/tests.

O 4. Discuss any special preoperative preparation procedures.

5. Identify the names and uses of ophthalmic instruments, supplies, and drugs.

6. Identify the names and uses of special equipment.

7. Discuss the intraoperative preparation of the patient undergoing an ophthalmic procedure.

8. Define and give an overview of the ophthalmic procedure.

9. Discuss the purpose and expected outcomes of the ophthalmic procedure.

10. Discuss the immediate postoperative care and possible complications of the ophthalmic procedure.

S 11. Discuss any specific variations related to the preoperative, intraoperative, and postoperative care of the ophthalmic patient.

CHAPTER 13

■ Key Terms

Define the following:

1. Anterior Chamber _____
   _____

2. BSS _____
   _____

3. Cataract _____
   _____

4. Chalazion _____
   _____

5. Dacryo- _____
   _____

6. Diathermy _____
   _____

7. Enucleation _____
   _____

8. Extracapsular Cataract Extraction _____
   _____

9. Extrinsic Muscles _____
   _____

10. Globe _____
    _____

11. Intracapsular Cataract Extraction _____
    _____

12. Intrinsic Muscles _____
    _____

13. Iridotomy _____
    _____

14. Kerato- _____
    _____

15. Lacrimal _____
    _____

16. Ocutome _____
    _____

17. O.D. _____
    _____

18. O.S. _____
    _____

19. O.U. _____
    _____

20. Posterior Chamber _____
    _____

21. Retrobulbar _____
    _____

22. Strabismus _____
    _____

23. Trephine _____
    _____

24. Tunic _____
    _____

25. Unilateral _____
    _____

■ Exercise A – Anatomy

1. Identify the structures of the eye shown in Figure 13-1.

Figure 13-1

Ophthalmic Surgery   173

A. _____
B. _____
C. _____
D. _____
E. _____
F. _____
G. _____
H. _____
I. _____
J. _____
K. _____
L. _____

2. Identify the nerves of the eye shown in Figure 13-2.

Figure 13-2

A. _____
B. _____
C. _____
D. _____
E. _____
F. _____
G. _____

3. Identify the muscles of the eye shown in Figure 13-3.

Figure 13-3

A. _____
B. _____
C. _____
D. _____
E. _____

4. Identify the structures of the lacrimal apparatus shown in Figure 13-4.

Figure 13-4

A. _____
B. _____

174 CHAPTER 13

C. _____
D. _____
E. _____
F. _____
G. _____
H. _____

5. Name the three tunics of the eye.

A. _____
B. _____
C. _____

6. Name the two intrinsic muscles of the eye.

A. _____
B. _____

7. Name the bones that form the orbit.

A. _____
B. _____
C. _____
D. _____
E. _____
F. _____
G. _____

8. Name the six extrinsic muscles of the eye and the primary function of each.

A. _____
B. _____
C. _____
D. _____
E. _____
F. _____

9. What are the four tissue layers that make up the cornea?

A. _____
B. _____

C. _____
D. _____

10. Vitreous humor fills the _____ chamber of the eye.

11. Briefly explain the process of accommodation.

_____
_____
_____
_____
_____

12. Describe the location of the crystalline lens.

_____
_____
_____
_____

13. List the refractive media of the eye.

A. _____
B. _____
C. _____
D. _____

14. What is the function of the iris? _____

_____
_____
_____
_____

15. Describe the functions of the rods and the cones.

_____
_____
_____
_____
_____

Exercise B – Pathology

1. Give three reasons for cataract formation.

   A. _____

   B. _____

   C. _____

2. Why is a cataract considered a condition rather than a disease? _____
_____
_____
_____

3. Describe what happens when a retinal detachment occurs. _____
_____
_____
_____

4. Explain why a patient may see "spots" or "flashes of light" with the development of a retinal detachment. _____
_____
_____
_____

5. What is a chalazion? _____
_____
_____
_____

6. Explain the difference between comitant and incomitant strabismus. _____
_____
_____
_____

7. List four causes of corneal clouding.

   A. _____

   B. _____

   C. _____

   D. _____

8. Name and describe the visual defect shown in Figure 13-5.

Figure 13-5

_____
_____
_____
_____

9. Name and describe the visual defect shown in Figure 13-6.

Figure 13-6

_____
_____
_____
_____

176 CHAPTER 13

10. Name and describe the visual defect shown in Figure 13-7.

Figure 13-7

_____
_____
_____
_____

11. Name and describe the visual defect shown in Figure 13-8.

Figure 13-8

_____
_____
_____
_____

12. What condition is characterized by excess pressure of the aqueous humor? _____
_____
_____
_____

13. What is an epiretinal membrane? _____
_____
_____
_____
_____
_____

14. List three indications for enucleation.

   A. _____
   B. _____
   C. _____

15. What visual deficit will occur in a person who lacks cones in the retina? _____
_____
_____
_____
_____
_____

■ Exercise C – Operation

1. How is intraocular pressure measured from within the sterile field? _____
_____
_____
_____
_____

2. What procedure is performed to open the blocked tear ducts of an infant? _____
_____
_____
_____
_____

3. List three methods for cataract extraction.

   A. _____
   B. _____
   C. _____

4. What is a diathermy apparatus used to accomplish? _____

5. How is cryotherapy used to treat retinal detachment? _____

6. Recession/resection is used for correction what condition of the eye? _____

7. What type of instrument is a trephine? In eye surgery, what is it used for? _____

8. What is the purpose of inserting a scleral buckle to treat retinal detachment? _____

9. List four complications that may arise following a scleral buckle procedure.

   A. _____

   B. _____

   C. _____

   D. _____

10. The topical anesthetic cocaine is often used to prepare the nose for dacryocystorhinostomy, even if a general anesthetic is planned. Why? _____

11. What is the main advantage of evisceration of the eye over enucleation? _____

12. What is sodium hyaluronate used for? _____

13. List the drapes necessary for surgery to expose the eye, and their order of application. _____

14. What is the purpose of applying fluorescein to the cornea? What tool must be used in conjunction with fluorescein? _____

15. What is the main advantage of phacoemulsification over traditional extracapsular cataract extraction? _____

Exercise D – Specific Variations

Student Name _____ Date _____

Instructor _____

Surgical Procedure – Student Case Study Report

The student will be provided with basic patient information (real or simulated) and is expected to complete the following case study.

1. Procedure name: _____
   _____
   _____

2. Definition of procedure: _____
   _____
   _____
   _____
   _____

3. What is the purpose of the procedure? _____
   _____
   _____
   _____
   _____

4. What is the expected outcome of the procedure?
   _____
   _____
   _____
   _____

5. Patient age: _____

6. Gender: _____

7. Additional pertinent patient information: _____
   _____
   _____
   _____

8. Probable preoperative diagnosis: _____
   _____
   _____
   _____
   _____
   _____
   _____

9. How was the diagnosis determined? _____
   _____
   _____
   _____
   _____

10. Discuss the relevant anatomy. _____
    _____
    _____
    _____
    _____
    _____

11. List the general and procedure-specific equipment that will be needed for the procedure.

    _____   _____
    _____   _____
    _____   _____
    _____   _____
    _____   _____
    _____   _____

Ophthalmic Surgery   179

12. List the general and procedure-specific instruments that will be needed for the procedure.

    _____   _____
    _____   _____
    _____   _____
    _____   _____
    _____   _____
    _____

13. List the basic and procedure-specific supplies that will be needed for the procedure.

    Pack _____
    Basin _____
    Gloves _____
    Blades _____
    Drapes _____
    _____
    Drains _____
    Dressings _____
    _____

    Suture – Type of Suture, Needle (if applicable), and Anticipated Tissue Usage

    _____   _____
    _____   _____
    _____   _____
    _____   _____
    _____   _____

    Pharmaceuticals

    _____   _____
    _____   _____
    _____   _____
    _____   _____
    _____   _____

    Miscellaneous

    _____   _____
    _____   _____
    _____   _____
    _____   _____
    _____   _____
    _____

14. Operative preparation: _____
    _____
    _____
    _____
    _____
    _____
    _____
    _____
    _____

15. What type of anesthesia will likely be used? Why?
    _____
    _____
    _____
    _____
    _____
    _____

16. List any special anesthesia equipment that may be needed. _____
    _____
    _____
    _____
    _____
    _____
    _____

17. Patient position during the procedure: _____
    _____
    _____
    _____
    _____

180   CHAPTER 13

18. What supplies will be necessary for positioning?
    _____
    _____
    _____
    _____
    _____

19. What type of shave/skin preparation will be necessary (if any)? _____
    _____
    _____
    _____
    _____

20. Define the anatomic perimeters of the prep.
    _____
    _____
    _____
    _____
    _____

21. List the order in which the drapes will be applied, and describe any specific variations.
    _____
    _____
    _____
    _____
    _____
    _____
    _____

22. List any practical considerations.
    _____
    _____
    _____
    _____
    _____

23. List the procedural steps, and describe the preparatory and supportive actions of the STSR during each step (use additional space if necessary).

Operative Procedure	Technical Considerations
1.	•
	•
2.	•
	•
3.	•
	•
4.	•
	•
5.	•
	•

Operative Procedure continued	**Technical Considerations** continued
6.	•
	•
7.	•
	•
8.	•
	•
9.	•
	•
10.	•
	•

24. What is the postoperative diagnosis? _____

25. Describe the immediate postoperative care.

26. What is the patient's long-term prognosis?

27. What are the possible complications? _____

28. Comments or questions: _____

29. What is the most valuable information you obtained from preparing this surgical procedure case study? _____

Case Studies

CASE STUDY 1

Susan is admitted to the hospital for eye surgery. She was diagnosed in childhood with diabetes and is now 50 years old. Susan also has been diagnosed with retinopathy, a frequent occurrence in diabetic patients. Her vision has been deteriorating over the last several years. She has recently suffered a vitreous hemorrhage due to neovascularization of the eye, which is common in diabetic patients.

1. What procedure will be performed to resolve the problem?

2. Briefly describe the procedure, and explain how Susan will benefit.

3. What are the two possible approaches the surgeon may use to enter the eye? Which is preferred?

4. What piece of equipment is crucial to a vitrectomy?

5. What substance, if any, will be used to replace the vitreous humor?

Ophthalmic Surgery   183

☐ CASE STUDY 2

Ronald has been having trouble with his stereoscopic vision. His wife says that he appears to have a "lazy eye." The amount of misalignment seems to stay the same no matter which direction his eyes are looking. Ronald has been admitted to the ambulatory care center for surgery.

1. What is the correct term for the condition that Ronald has?

2. Would this condition be considered "comitant" or "incomitant?"

3. What surgical procedure will be performed to correct this condition?

4. In which position will Ronald be placed for this procedure?

5. What are the anatomic boundaries for the prep?

CHAPTER 14

Otorhinolaryngologic Surgery

OBJECTIVES

After studying this chapter, the reader should be able to:

A 1. Discuss the relevant anatomy of the ear, nose, and upper aerodigestive tract.

P 2. Describe the pathology that prompts otorhinolaryngologic surgical intervention and the related terminology.

3. Discuss any special preoperative otorhinolaryngologic diagnostic procedures/tests.

O 4. Discuss any special otorhinolaryngologic preoperative preparation procedures.

5. Identify the names and uses of otorhinolaryngologic instruments, supplies, and drugs.

6. Identify the names and uses of special otorhinolaryngologic equipment.

7. Discuss the intraoperative preparation of the patient undergoing an otorhinolaryngologic procedure.

8. Define and give an overview of the otorhinolaryngologic procedure.

9. Discuss the purpose and expected outcomes of the otorhinolaryngologic procedure.

10. Discuss the immediate postoperative care and possible complications of the otorhinolaryngologic procedure.

S 11. Discuss any specific variations related to the preoperative, intraoperative, and postoperative care of the otorhinolaryngologic patient.

CHAPTER 14

■ Key Terms

Define the following:

1. Aerodigestive Tract
2. Apnea
3. Carina
4. Cholesteatoma
5. Congenital
6. Dynamic Equilibrium
7. Epiglottis
8. Epistaxis
9. Gelfoam
10. Glottis
11. Hydrops
12. Hypertrophy
13. Laryngo-
14. Myringo-
15. Olfaction
16. Oropharynx
17. Oto-
18. Polyp
19. Polysomnography
20. Pharyngotympanic tube
21. Rhino-
22. Sclerosis
23. SMR
24. T&A
25. UPPP

Exercise A – Anatomy

1. Identify the structures of the ear shown in Figure 14-1.

   A. _____   B. _____
   C. _____   D. _____
   E. _____   F. _____
   G. _____   H. _____

2. Identify the structures of the upper aerodigestive tract shown in Figure 14-2.

   A. _____   B. _____
   C. _____   D. _____
   E. _____   F. _____
   G. _____   H. _____
   I. _____   J. _____
   K. _____   L. _____
   M. _____   N. _____
   O. _____   P. _____
   Q. _____

Figure 14-2

Figure 14-1

188 CHAPTER 14

Figure 14-3

3. Identify the structures shown in Figure 14-3.

   A. _____

   B. _____

   C. _____

   D. _____

   E. _____

   F. _____

   G. _____

4. List two functions of the nose.

   A. _____
   _____

   B. _____
   _____

5. Which bone houses the mastoid sinus? _____
   _____
   _____
   _____

6. Name the three sections of the pharynx. _____

   A. _____

   B. _____

   C. _____

7. Which of the tonsils are removed during a tonsillectomy? _____
   _____
   _____
   _____
   _____

8. Name the four pairs of paranasal sinuses, and give their locations.

   A. _____

   B. _____

   C. _____

   D. _____

9. How many layers comprise the tympanic membrane, and what is the composition of each layer?
   _____
   _____
   _____
   _____

10. Where would you find the umbo and cone of light, and what are they? _____

11. Provide the scientific and common names for the ossicles in their proper sequence, moving from lateral to medial. _____

12. How many nasal bones does each individual normally have, and what is their function? _____

13. What are nasal conchae, and describe their function? _____

14. What is the main source of arterial blood to the nose, and from which vessel is it derived? _____

15. Where are the adenoids located? _____

■ Exercise B – Pathology

1. Can tonsillitis affect the palatine tonsils? _____

2. Which nerve is affected in a patient with sensorineural deafness? _____

3. What is the cause of hypertrophied turbinates? _____

4. What is the cause of obstructive sleep apnea? _____

5. What is the most common cause of otitis media? _____

6. What causes the nasal septum to deviate from the midline? _____

CHAPTER 14

7. Where is a Zenker's diverticulum located, and which diagnostic exam will be helpful in determining the diagnosis? _____

8. List the symptoms of Ménière's syndrome.

9. List several reasons for nasal septal perforation.

10. What is the most frequent cause of epiglottitis?

11. Swimmer's ear is a specific example of what more general condition? _____

12. What are some of the causes of nasal obstruction?

13. What is the usual cause of a vocal cord nodule?

14. Define deafness. _____

15. What is the origin of a polyp? _____

■ Exercise C – Operation

1. What is the name of the procedure used to remove nasal polyps, and what special instrument may be used to perform the procedure?

2. What is the unique feature of the #12 knife blade?

3. Are any special precautions necessary when using a carbon dioxide laser? If so, what are they?

4. Describe the differences between rhinoplasty and septoplasty.

5. Which tonsils are typically removed during a tonsillectomy?

6. What are the reasons for reversing the operating table during ear surgery?

7. Is sinus endoscopy a diagnostic or a functional procedure? Why?

8. An adult patient undergoing tonsillectomy with local anesthesia will be placed in what position?

9. What source of energy will be needed to operate the rotating drill?

10. What is intranasal antrostomy, and what special instrument may be needed to facilitate the procedure?

11. What is the most common autologous site for securing a graft for myringoplasty?

12. What are the classifications for tympanoplasty, and how are they determined?

13. Where is the incision made to facilitate drainage of the frontal sinus? _____

14. What is the pillar dissector used for? _____

15. Describe panendoscopy, and list any special equipment that may be required. _____

Exercise D – Specific Variations

Student Name _____ Date _____

Instructor _____

Surgical Procedure – Student Case Study Report

The student will be provided with basic patient information (real or simulated) and is expected to complete the following case study.

1. Procedure name: _____
   _____
   _____

2. Definition of procedure: _____
   _____
   _____
   _____

3. What is the purpose of the procedure? _____
   _____
   _____
   _____

4. What is the expected outcome of the procedure?
   _____
   _____
   _____
   _____

5. Patient age: _____

6. Gender: _____

7. Additional pertinent patient information: _____
   _____
   _____
   _____

8. Probable preoperative diagnosis: _____
   _____
   _____
   _____
   _____

9. How was the diagnosis determined? _____
   _____
   _____
   _____
   _____

10. Discuss the relevant anatomy. _____
    _____
    _____
    _____
    _____
    _____

11. List the general and procedure-specific equipment that will be needed for the procedure.

    _____   _____
    _____   _____
    _____   _____
    _____   _____
    _____   _____

194 CHAPTER 14

12. List the general and procedure-specific instruments that will be needed for the procedure.

    _____   _____
    _____   _____
    _____   _____
    _____   _____
    _____   _____
    _____   _____

13. List the basic and procedure-specific supplies that will be needed for the procedure.

    Pack _____
    Basin _____
    Gloves _____
    Blades _____
    Drapes _____
    _____
    Drains _____
    Dressings _____
    _____

    Suture – Type of Suture, Needle (if applicable), and Anticipated Tissue Usage

    _____   _____
    _____   _____
    _____   _____
    _____   _____
    _____   _____

    Pharmaceuticals

    _____   _____
    _____   _____
    _____   _____
    _____   _____

Miscellaneous

_____   _____
_____   _____
_____   _____
_____   _____
_____   _____
_____   _____

14. Operative preparation: _____
    _____
    _____
    _____
    _____
    _____
    _____

15. What type of anesthesia will likely be used? Why?
    _____
    _____
    _____
    _____
    _____
    _____

16. List any special anesthesia equipment that may be needed. _____
    _____
    _____
    _____
    _____
    _____

17. Patient position during the procedure: _____
    _____
    _____
    _____
    _____

18. What supplies will be necessary for positioning? _____

19. What type of shave/skin preparation will be necessary (if any)? _____

20. Define the anatomic perimeters of the prep. _____

21. List the order in which the drapes will be applied, and describe any specific variations. _____

22. List any practical considerations. _____

23. List the procedural steps, and describe the preparatory and supportive actions of the STSR during each step (use additional space if necessary).

Operative Procedure	Technical Considerations
1.	• •
2.	• •
3.	• •
4.	• •
5.	• •

CHAPTER 14

Operative Procedure *continued*	Technical Considerations *continued*
6.	•
	•
7.	•
	•
8.	•
	•
9.	•
	•
10.	•
	•

24. What is the postoperative diagnosis? _____

25. Describe the immediate postoperative care.

26. What is the patient's long-term prognosis?

27. What are the possible complications? _____

28. Comments or questions: _____

29. What is the most valuable information you obtained from preparing this surgical procedure case study? _____

Case Studies

CASE STUDY 1

Stan, a 46-year-old male, is about to spend the night in the "sleep lab." After numerous complaints from his wife that his heavy snoring is keeping her awake, Stan visited his primary care physician. Following a complete physical, Stan has been diagnosed with hypertension and obesity, and he was referred to an otorhinolaryngologist.

1. What tests will Stan undergo in the "sleep lab"? _____

2. What diagnosis do you think that the otorhinolaryngologist is considering? _____

3. What are Stan's conservative treatment options? _____

4. If Stan's condition eventually requires surgery, which procedure will be performed, and what structures will be removed? _____

CASE STUDY 2

Fred, a 4-year-old male, has been placed in respite foster care because of his uncontrollable temper tantrums, which include long bouts of screaming. The foster family noticed that Fred's voice was hoarse and that it did not improve over time. He was seen by an otorhinolaryngologist, who determined that Fred has developed nodules on his vocal cords.

1. Is Fred's condition life-threatening? _____

2. How was Fred's condition diagnosed? _____

3. What action will be necessary to treat Fred's condition? _____

4. If surgery is required, what type of procedure will be necessary, and how will it be accomplished?

5. If surgery is necessary, will the foster parents have the legal authority to sign his operative consent?

CHAPTER 15

Oral and Maxillofacial Surgery

OBJECTIVES

After studying this chapter, the reader should be able to:

A 1. Discuss the anatomy relevant to oral and maxillofacial surgery.

P 2. Describe the pathology that prompts oral and maxillofacial surgery and the related terminology.

3. Discuss any special preoperative diagnostic procedures/tests pertaining to oral and maxillofacial surgery.

O 4. Discuss special preoperative preparation procedures related to oral and maxillofacial surgery.

5. Identify the names and uses of oral and maxillofacial instruments, supplies, and drugs.

6. Identify the names and uses of special equipment used for oral and maxillofacial surgery.

7. Discuss the intraoperative preparation of the patient undergoing an oral or maxillofacial procedure.

8. Define and give an overview of oral or maxillofacial procedures.

9. Discuss the purpose and expected outcomes of oral and maxillofacial procedures.

10. Discuss the immediate postoperative care and possible complications of oral and maxillofacial procedures.

S 11. Discuss any specific variations related to the preoperative, intraoperative, and postoperative care of the oral and maxillofacial surgical patient.

CHAPTER 15

■ Key Terms

Define the following:

1. Alveolar Process _____

2. Arthroplasty _____

3. Arthroscopy _____

4. Arthrotomy _____

5. Bite Block _____

6. Calvarial _____

7. Condyle _____

8. Coronal Flap _____

9. Craniosynostosis _____

10. Dentition _____

11. Glenoid Fossa _____

12. -gnath _____

13. Labia _____

14. Malar Bone _____

15. Malocclusion _____

16. Maxillofacial _____

17. Meniscus _____

18. Orbicular _____

19. Osteotomy _____

20. Pan- _____

21. Ramus _____

22. Reduction _____

23. Sagittal _____

24. Symphysis _____

25. TMJ _____

Oral and Maxillofacial Surgery

■ Exercise A – Anatomy

1. Identify the bones of the anterior skull shown in Figure 15-1.

   A. _____
   B. _____
   C. _____
   D. _____
   E. _____
   F. _____
   G. _____
   H. _____

2. Identify the structures of the lateral skull shown in Figure 15-2.

   A. _____
   B. _____
   C. _____
   D. _____
   E. _____
   F. _____
   G. _____
   H. _____
   I. _____
   J. _____
   K. _____
   L. _____
   M. _____

Figure 15-1

Figure 15-2

202   CHAPTER 15

Figure 15-3

Figure 15-4

3. Identify the structures of the mouth shown in Figure 15-3.

   A. _____
   B. _____
   C. _____
   D. _____
   E. _____
   F. _____
   G. _____
   H. _____
   I. _____
   J. _____
   K. _____
   L. _____
   M. _____
   N. _____

4. Identify the bones of the orbit shown in Figure 15-4.

   A. _____
   B. _____
   C. _____
   D. _____
   E. _____
   F. _____
   G. _____
   H. _____
   I. _____
   J. _____

5. The anterior portion of the palate is referred to as the _____ palate.

6. What is the location and function of the soft palate? _____
   _____
   _____
   _____
   _____

7. The malar bone is also referred to as the _____ bone.

8. What are the inferior nasal conchae, and what is their function? _____

9. What is another name for the facial nerve? Which facial muscles are innervated by the facial nerve? _____

10. Which four muscles control movement of the lower jaw? _____

11. When does embryologic development of the face occur? _____

12. Where is the orbicularis oris muscle situated? What is its function? _____

13. Describe the components and features of the TMJ. _____

14. What is the ramus of the mandible? _____

15. What are the two main functions of the orbit? _____

■ Exercise B – Pathology

1. What are dental caries, and what is their cause? _____

2. What is meant by the term malocclusion? List two causes. _____

3. How does Paget's disease affect facial anatomy? _____

4. Describe a tri-malar fracture. _____

_____

_____

_____

_____

5. List the four categories of mandibular fractures.

   A. _____

   B. _____

   C. _____

   D. _____

6. What type of midfacial fracture is the most common? _____

_____

_____

_____

7. What is laterognathism? List two causes. _____

_____

_____

   A. _____

   B. _____

8. What specific radiographic view is used to detect a fracture of the frontal bone? _____

_____

_____

_____

9. Define cerebrospinal rhinorrhea. _____

_____

_____

_____

10. List three methods for diagnosing a zygomatic fracture. _____

_____

_____

_____

_____

11. List three visual findings that could indicate the presence of a zygomatic fracture.

    A. _____

    B. _____

    C. _____

12. Premature closure of the sutures of the skull is called _____.

13. Name and describe the four categories of tooth fractures.

    A. _____

    B. _____

    C. _____

    D. _____

14. List two advantages of three-dimensional imaging.

    A. _____

    B. _____

15. In addition to radiographic studies (including three-dimensional imaging), what other items may be useful to the surgeon during facial reconstruction surgery? _____

_____

_____

_____

_____

Exercise C – Operation

1. What is the importance of having the X-rays in the operating room prior to and during the surgical procedure? _____

2. What is accomplished by inserting a bite block during certain oral surgical procedures? _____

3. What is the purpose of inserting a throat pack? How is it inserted? _____

4. When is the throat pack removed? Why? _____

5. List two options for sealing an intranasal dural tear.
   A. _____
   B. _____

6. Define "autogenous", and list two possible donor sites for autogenous bone grafts. _____
   A. _____
   B. _____

7. Why is a local anesthetic with epinephrine often injected at the operative site preoperatively when the patient is under general anesthesia? _____

8. Describe the location of a coronal incision. _____

9. List two methods for securing a soft tissue flap in position.
   A. _____
   B. _____

10. In what position will the patient be placed for a posterior cranial expansion? _____

11. What type of procedure is performed to treat orthognathia? _____

12. What can be done during lengthy oral procedures to prevent drying and cracking of the lips? _____

13. Why is it important to assure that all metal implants are of the same type?

14. If a bone graft is needed during a procedure in which the patient has a coronal incision, what type of bone will be considered as the first choice? Why?

15. In what situation(s) is arch bar fixation employed?

Oral and Maxillofacial Surgery   207

■ Exercise D – Specific Variations

Student Name _____ Date _____

Instructor _____

Surgical Procedure – Student Case Study Report

The student will be provided with basic patient information (real or simulated) and is expected to complete the following case study.

1. Procedure name: _____
   _____
   _____

2. Definition of procedure: _____
   _____
   _____
   _____
   _____

3. What is the purpose of the procedure? _____
   _____
   _____
   _____
   _____

4. What is the expected outcome of the procedure?
   _____
   _____
   _____
   _____

5. Patient age: _____

6. Gender: _____

7. Additional pertinent patient information: _____
   _____
   _____
   _____

8. Probable preoperative diagnosis: _____
   _____
   _____
   _____
   _____
   _____

9. How was the diagnosis determined? _____
   _____
   _____
   _____
   _____
   _____

10. Discuss the relevant anatomy. _____
    _____
    _____
    _____
    _____
    _____

11. List the general and procedure-specific equipment that will be needed for the procedure.
    _____   _____
    _____   _____
    _____   _____
    _____   _____
    _____   _____

CHAPTER 15

12. List the general and procedure-specific instruments that will be needed for the procedure.

   _____ _____
   _____ _____
   _____ _____
   _____ _____
   _____ _____
   _____ _____

13. List the basic and procedure-specific supplies that will be needed for the procedure.

   Pack _____

   Basin _____

   Gloves _____

   Blades _____

   Drapes _____
   _____

   Drains _____

   Dressings _____
   _____

   Suture – Type of Suture, Needle (if applicable), and Anticipated Tissue Usage

   _____ _____
   _____ _____
   _____ _____
   _____ _____
   _____ _____

   Pharmaceuticals

   _____ _____
   _____ _____
   _____ _____
   _____ _____

Miscellaneous

   _____ _____
   _____ _____
   _____ _____
   _____ _____
   _____ _____
   _____ _____

14. Operative preparation: _____
   _____
   _____
   _____
   _____
   _____
   _____
   _____

15. What type of anesthesia will likely be used? Why?
   _____
   _____
   _____
   _____
   _____
   _____

16. List any special anesthesia equipment that may be needed. _____
   _____
   _____
   _____
   _____
   _____
   _____

17. Patient position during the procedure: _____
   _____
   _____
   _____

18. What supplies will be necessary for positioning?
   _____
   _____
   _____
   _____

19. What type of shave/skin preparation will be necessary (if any)? _____
   _____
   _____
   _____
   _____

20. Define the anatomic perimeters of the prep.
   _____
   _____
   _____
   _____
   _____

21. List the order in which the drapes will be applied, and describe any specific variations.
   _____
   _____
   _____
   _____
   _____
   _____
   _____

22. List any practical considerations.
   _____
   _____
   _____
   _____
   _____

23. List the procedural steps, and describe the preparatory and supportive actions of the STSR during each step (use additional space if necessary).

Operative Procedure	Technical Considerations
1.	•
	•
2.	•
	•
3.	•
	•
4.	•
	•
5.	•
	•

Operative Procedure continued	**Technical Considerations** continued
6.	•
	•
7.	•
	•
8.	•
	•
9.	•
	•
10.	•
	•

24. What is the postoperative diagnosis? _____
_____
_____
_____
_____

25. Describe the immediate postoperative care.
_____
_____
_____
_____
_____

26. What is the patient's long-term prognosis?
_____
_____
_____
_____
_____

27. What are the possible complications? _____
_____
_____
_____
_____

28. Comments or questions: _____
_____
_____
_____
_____

29. What is the most valuable information you obtained from preparing this surgical procedure case study? _____
_____
_____
_____

Case Studies

CASE STUDY 1

Lucricia is a 14-year-old with cerebral palsy and epilepsy. She is scheduled for dental restoration, including gingivectomy for hyperplasia of her gums, under general anesthesia.

1. What procedures may be performed during dental restoration?

2. Why is general anesthesia indicated in Lucricia's case?

3. What is the most likely reason that Lucricia suffers from hyperplasia of her gums that is severe enough to require gingivectomy?

CASE STUDY 2

Roberto experienced a severe blow to his left cheek when he accidentally struck the corner of the wall as he was rushing through a dark hallway during the night, on his way to the bathroom. He is suffering severe pain, and it appears to him that his face no longer has a symmetrical appearance.

1. What type of injury do you suspect that Roberto has incurred? _____

2. What type of examination(s) will be performed by the maxillofacial surgeon to confirm the diagnosis?

3. How will Roberto's problem be corrected? _____

Plastic and Reconstructive Surgery

CHAPTER 16

OBJECTIVES

After studying this chapter, the reader should be able to:

A 1. Discuss the relevant anatomy and physiology of the skin and its underlying tissues.

P 2. Describe the pathology that prompts plastic/reconstructive surgical intervention and the related terminology.

3. Discuss any special preoperative plastic/reconstructive diagnostic procedures/tests.

O 4. Discuss any special preoperative preparation procedures related to plastic/reconstructive surgical procedures.

5. Identify the names and uses of plastic/reconstructive instruments, supplies, and drugs.

6. Identify the names and uses of any special equipment related to plastic/reconstructive surgery.

7. Discuss the intraoperative preparation of the patient undergoing a plastic/reconstructive procedure.

8. Define and give an overview of the plastic/reconstructive procedure.

9. Discuss the purpose and expected outcomes of the plastic/reconstructive procedure.

10. Discuss the immediate postoperative care and possible complications of the plastic/reconstructive procedure.

S 11. Discuss any specific variations related to the preoperative, intraoperative, and postoperative care of the plastic/reconstructive patient.

CHAPTER 16

■ Key Terms

Define the following:

1. Aesthetics _____
2. Arthrodesis _____
3. Augmentation _____
4. Carpal Tunnel _____
5. Cheilo- _____
6. Cleft _____
7. Dermatome _____
8. Elliptical _____
9. Ganglion Cyst _____
10. Gynecomastia _____
11. Integument _____
12. MPJ _____
13. Neurorrhaphy _____
14. Panniculus _____
15. Poly- _____
16. Radial Hypoplasia _____
17. Replantation _____
18. Rhinoplasty _____
19. -schisis _____
20. Sebum _____
21. STSG _____
22. Syndactyly _____
23. Synthesis _____
24. Triquetrum _____
25. Xenograft _____

Plastic and Reconstructive Surgery 215

Exercise A – Anatomy

1. Identify the structures shown in Figure 16-1.

   A. _____
   B. _____
   C. _____
   D. _____
   E. _____
   F. _____
   G. _____
   H. _____
   I. _____
   J. _____
   K. _____
   L. _____
   M. _____
   N. _____
   O. _____
   P. _____
   Q. _____

2. Identify the bones of the dorsal hand shown in Figure 16-2.

   A. _____
   B. _____
   C. _____
   D. _____
   E. _____
   F. _____
   G. _____
   H. _____
   I. _____
   J. _____
   K. _____
   L. _____
   M. _____
   N. _____
   O. _____
   P. _____

Figure 16-1

Figure 16-2

216   CHAPTER 16

6. List the major functions of the skin.

   A. _____
   B. _____
   C. _____
   D. _____
   E. _____
   F. _____
   G. _____

7. Sweat glands are also known as the _____ glands.

8. Name and briefly describe the three types of sudoriferous glands.

   A. _____
   _____
   B. _____
   _____
   C. _____
   _____

Figure 16-3

3. Identify the nasal structures shown in Figure 16-3.

   A. _____
   B. _____
   C. _____
   D. _____
   E. _____

9. Name the structures that are contained in the anterior (palmar) compartment of the hand.

   _____
   _____
   _____
   _____

4. Identify the structures of the breast shown in Figure 16-4.

   A. _____
   B. _____
   C. _____
   D. _____
   E. _____
   F. _____
   G. _____

5. Name the two major layers of the integumentary system.

   A. _____
   B. _____

Figure 16-4

10. Development of the upper limb is complete by the _____ week in utero.

11. Name the five layers of the epidermis in sequence from outermost to innermost layer.

    A. _____

    B. _____

    C. _____

    D. _____

    E. _____

12. Name the three functions of the subcutaneous tissue layer.

    A. _____

    B. _____

    C. _____

13. Name the two divisions of the dermis, and briefly describe them.

    A. _____

    B. _____

14. Name the secretion that is produced in the sebaceous glands. What is the purpose of the secretion? _____
    _____
    _____
    _____
    _____

15. What is the function of the palate? _____
    _____
    _____
    _____
    _____

Exercise B – Pathology

1. Which tissue layer(s) is/are affected by a second-degree burn? _____
   _____
   _____
   _____

2. Use the Rule of Nines to determine the percentage of the body surface area affected by a third-degree burn of the chest, back, and left arm.
   _____
   _____
   _____
   _____

3. Name the bacteria that are the main causative agents of acne vulgaris.

   A. _____

   B. _____

   C. _____

4. Only 20% of cleft deformities are genetic. What is/are the cause(s) of the remaining 80%? _____
   _____
   _____
   _____
   _____

5. What is the most common type of polydactyly?
   _____
   _____
   _____
   _____

6. What is a ganglion cyst? _____
   _____
   _____
   _____
   _____

7. What causes the formation of a ganglion cyst?

8. Name three treatment options for a ganglion cyst.

   A.

   B.

   C.

9. What is the cause of ptosis of the eyelid? _____

10. Define neoplasm. Is a neoplasm malignant?

11. Give three examples of common malignant neoplasms of the skin.

    A.

    B.

    C.

12. What is the cause of cheiloschisis and palatoschisis? _____

13. Name two diseases of the hand that are caused by stenosing tenosynovitis.

    A.

    B.

14. List two manifestations of palmar fascia contraction (Dupuytren's disease).

    A.

    B.

15. What is the cause of rheumatoid arthritis? _____

Exercise C – Operation

1. Describe the difference between nasal and rhinoplasty instrumentation. _____

2. What is the purpose/function of a dermatome?

3. List two possible power sources for the oscillating-blade-type dermatome.

   A.

   B.

4. What is the purpose of a mesh graft device?

5. What is the purpose of a tacking suture?

6. What is the advantage of tumescent liposuction over the traditional method?

7. What is the common name for the umbilical template used during abdominoplasty? What is its purpose?

8. How is sterile mineral oil used during procurement of a STSG?

9. How is the recipient site prepared prior to placement of a STSG? Why?

10. Why is palatoplasty considered a clean, rather than sterile, procedure?

11. What anatomic area is prepped prior to draping for hand surgery?

12. Why is the extremity wrapped with an Esmarch prior to tourniquet inflation?

13. Provide two indications for joint replacement in the hand.

   A.

   B.

14. Replantation of a digit begins with the attachment of which structure(s)?

15. List four incision options that are used to achieve augmentation mammoplasty by producing a minimal or completely hidden scar.

   A.

   B.

   C.

   D.

Exercise D – Specific Variations

Student Name _____ Date _____

Instructor _____

Surgical Procedure – Student Case Study Report

The student will be provided with basic patient information (real or simulated) and is expected to complete the following case study.

1. Procedure name: _____
   _____
   _____

2. Definition of procedure: _____
   _____
   _____
   _____

3. What is the purpose of the procedure? _____
   _____
   _____
   _____

4. What is the expected outcome of the procedure?
   _____
   _____
   _____
   _____

5. Patient age: _____
6. Gender: _____
7. Additional pertinent patient information: _____
   _____
   _____

8. Probable preoperative diagnosis: _____
   _____
   _____
   _____
   _____
   _____

9. How was the diagnosis determined? _____
   _____
   _____
   _____
   _____

10. Discuss the relevant anatomy. _____
    _____
    _____
    _____
    _____
    _____

11. List the general and procedure-specific equipment that will be needed for the procedure.
    _____ _____
    _____ _____
    _____ _____
    _____ _____
    _____ _____

12. List the general and procedure-specific instruments that will be needed for the procedure.

   _____ _____
   _____ _____
   _____ _____
   _____ _____
   _____ _____
   _____ _____

13. List the basic and procedure-specific supplies that will be needed for the procedure.

   Pack _____
   Basin _____
   Gloves _____
   Blades _____
   Drapes _____
   _____
   Drains _____
   Dressings _____
   _____

   Suture – Type of Suture, Needle (if applicable), and Anticipated Tissue Usage

   _____ _____
   _____ _____
   _____ _____
   _____ _____
   _____ _____
   _____ _____

   Pharmaceuticals

   _____ _____
   _____ _____
   _____ _____
   _____ _____

   Miscellaneous

   _____ _____
   _____ _____
   _____ _____
   _____ _____
   _____ _____
   _____ _____

14. Operative preparation: _____
    _____
    _____
    _____
    _____
    _____
    _____
    _____

15. What type of anesthesia will likely be used? Why?
    _____
    _____
    _____
    _____
    _____
    _____

16. List any special anesthesia equipment that may be needed. _____
    _____
    _____
    _____
    _____
    _____
    _____
    _____

17. Patient position during the procedure: _____
    _____
    _____
    _____
    _____
    _____

222 CHAPTER 16

18. What supplies will be necessary for positioning?

_____

_____

_____

_____

19. What type of shave/skin preparation will be necessary (if any)? _____

_____

_____

_____

_____

20. Define the anatomic perimeters of the prep.

_____

_____

_____

_____

21. List the order in which the drapes will be applied, and describe any specific variations.

_____

_____

_____

_____

_____

_____

22. List any practical considerations.

_____

_____

_____

_____

_____

23. List the procedural steps, and describe the preparatory and supportive actions of the STSR during each step (use additional space if necessary).

Operative Procedure	Technical Considerations
1.	•
	•
2.	•
	•
3.	•
	•
4.	•
	•
5.	•
	•

Plastic and Reconstructive Surgery 223

Operative Procedure *continued*	Technical Considerations *continued*
6.	•
	•
7.	•
	•
8.	•
	•
9.	•
	•
10.	•
	•

24. What is the postoperative diagnosis? _____

25. Describe the immediate postoperative care.

26. What is the patient's long-term prognosis?

27. What are the possible complications? _____

28. Comments or questions: _____

29. What is the most valuable information you obtained from preparing this surgical procedure case study? _____

Case Studies

CASE STUDY 1

Three-year-old Bobby accidentally pulled on the tablecloth, causing his mother's scalding coffee to spill on his left neck, shoulder, and chest. It has been determined that Bobby has suffered second- and third-degree burns over 9% of his body. The accident occurred three weeks ago, and Bobby is now scheduled for a STSG.

1. How was the extent of Bobby's injury determined? _____

2. What was the biggest risk that Bobby faced with these third-degree burns? _____

3. What is "STSG," and what special instrument will be required to obtain the graft? _____

4. From which anatomic site is the graft most likely to be procured? _____

CASE STUDY 2

Sven is a 62-year-old dairy farmer. He has been diagnosed with Dupuytren's disease. The disease has progressed to the point where Sven is unable to use his right hand effectively to connect the milking machine to his cows. He has put off surgery as long as possible, but now the inevitable has arrived.

1. What is Dupuytren's disease?

   _____
   _____
   _____
   _____

2. Is the condition painful?

   _____
   _____
   _____
   _____

3. What procedure will be necessary to treat Sven's condition?

   _____
   _____
   _____
   _____

4. Can Sven expect to regain full function and normal appearance?

   _____
   _____
   _____
   _____

CHAPTER 17

Genitourinary Surgery

OBJECTIVES

After studying this chapter, the reader should be able to:

A 1. Discuss the relevant anatomy of the genitourinary system.

P 2. Describe the pathology that prompts genitourinary system surgical intervention and the related terminology.

3. Discuss any special preoperative genitourinary diagnostic procedures/tests.

O 4. Discuss any special preoperative genitourinary preparation procedures.

5. Identify the names and uses of genitourinary instruments, supplies, and drugs.

6. Identify the names and uses of special genitourinary equipment.

7. Discuss the intraoperative preparation of the patient undergoing the genitourinary procedure.

8. Define and give an overview of the genitourinary procedure.

9. Discuss the purpose and expected outcomes of the genitourinary procedure.

10. Discuss the immediate postoperative care and possible complications of the genitourinary procedure.

S 11. Discuss any specific variations related to the preoperative, intraoperative, and postoperative care of the genitourinary patient.

CHAPTER 17

■ Key Terms

Define the following:

1. ACTH _____
2. Afferent _____
3. Calculi _____
4. Conduit _____
5. Cortex _____
6. ESWL _____
7. Focal Point _____
8. Gerota's Fascia _____
9. Gibson Incision _____
10. Hilum _____
11. Hirsutism _____
12. Hypertrophy _____
13. Hypospadias _____
14. Incontinence _____
15. Intravenous Urogram _____
16. Medulla _____
17. Prepuce _____
18. Retroperitoneal _____
19. Rugae _____
20. Stoma _____
21. Suprarenal Glands _____
22. Torsion _____
23. TURP _____
24. UTI _____
25. Vesical _____

Genitourinary Surgery 229

Exercise A – Anatomy

1. Identify the structures shown in Figure 17-1.

   A. _____
   B. _____
   C. _____
   D. _____
   E. _____
   F. _____
   G. _____
   H. _____
   I. _____
   J. _____
   K. _____
   L. _____
   M. _____
   N. _____
   O. _____
   P. _____
   Q. _____
   R. _____

Figure 17-1

230   CHAPTER 17

Figure 17-2

Figure 17-3

2. Identify the structures shown in Figure 17-2.

   A. _____
   B. _____
   C. _____
   D. _____
   E. _____
   F. _____
   G. _____

3. Identify the structures shown in Figure 17-3.

   A. _____
   B. _____
   C. _____
   D. _____
   E. _____
   F. _____
   G. _____
   H. _____

Genitourinary Surgery   231

Figure 17-4

Figure 17-5

4. Identify the structures shown in Figure 17-4.

   A. _____
   B. _____
   C. _____
   D. _____
   E. _____
   F. _____
   G. _____
   H. _____
   I. _____
   J. _____

5. Identify the structures shown in Figure 17-5.

   A. _____
   B. _____
   C. _____
   D. _____
   E. _____
   F. _____
   G. _____
   H. _____
   I. _____
   J. _____

232　CHAPTER 17

K. _____
L. _____
M. _____
N. _____
O. _____
P. _____
Q. _____
R. _____
S. _____
T. _____

6. Identify the structures of the testis shown in Figure 17-6.

A. _____
B. _____
C. _____
D. _____
E. _____

F. _____
G. _____
H. _____
I. _____
J. _____
K. _____
L. _____

7. Trace the pathway that sperm cells follow through the ducts of the male reproductive system by placing the following elements in the correct order.

A. _____ Ductus deferens
B. _____ Ejaculatory duct
C. _____ Epididymis
D. _____ Seminiferous tubules (testis)
E. _____ Urethra

8. Trace the pathway of fluid from the time it leaves the circulatory system until it leaves the body as urine by placing the following elements in the correct order.

A. _____ Afferent arteriole
B. _____ Bladder
C. _____ Bowman's capsule
D. _____ Calyx
E. _____ Collecting tubule
F. _____ Distal convoluted tubule
G. _____ Glomerulus
H. _____ Loop of Henle
I. _____ Proximal convoluted tubule
J. _____ Renal artery
K. _____ Renal pelvis
L. _____ Ureter
M. _____ Urethra

Figure 17-6

2. List at least three features of the Cysto Room that may not be found in the general OR. _____

_____

_____

_____

_____

3. What is the function of a deflecting mechanism?

_____

_____

_____

_____

4. What is the purpose of an O'Connor shield?

_____

_____

_____

_____

5. What specific structure is the Gibson incision designed to access? _____

_____

_____

_____

6. In which position is the patient placed when use of a flank incision is anticipated? _____

_____

_____

_____

7. List the three flank incision options and give a brief description of the location of each.

A. _____

_____

B. _____

_____

C. _____

_____

8. What is the purpose of renal cooling?

_____

_____

_____

_____

9. Why is it important for the STSR to have a chest tube, insertion supplies, and a water-seal drainage system readily available during a nephrectomy?

_____

_____

_____

_____

_____

10. List the three sources from which kidneys are obtained for transplant.

A. _____

B. _____

C. _____

11. What is the purpose of suprapubic cystostomy?

_____

_____

_____

12. Will the surgical technologist be scrubbed in for cystoscopy? What is the main function of the surgical technologist during cystoscopy? _____
_____
_____
_____

13. List four procedures that may be performed transurethrally.

   A. _____
   B. _____
   C. _____
   D. _____

14. Why is it necessary for the assistant to change the gloves (and possibly the gown) during MMK?
_____
_____
_____
_____

15. What is the purpose of repeatedly introducing the cystoscope during a Stamey procedure? _____
_____
_____
_____
_____

Exercise D – Specific Variations

Student Name _____ Date _____

Instructor _____

Surgical Procedure – Student Case Study Report

The student will be provided with basic patient information (real or simulated) and is expected to complete the following case study.

1. Procedure name: _____
   _____
   _____

2. Definition of procedure: _____
   _____
   _____
   _____

3. What is the purpose of the procedure? _____
   _____
   _____
   _____

4. What is the expected outcome of the procedure?
   _____
   _____
   _____

5. Patient age: _____
6. Gender: _____
7. Additional pertinent patient information: _____
   _____
   _____

8. Probable preoperative diagnosis: _____
   _____
   _____
   _____
   _____

9. How was the diagnosis determined? _____
   _____
   _____
   _____
   _____

10. Discuss the relevant anatomy. _____
    _____
    _____
    _____
    _____

11. List the general and procedure-specific equipment that will be needed for the procedure.

    _____ _____
    _____ _____
    _____ _____
    _____ _____
    _____ _____
    _____ _____

12. List the general and procedure-specific instruments that will be needed for the procedure.

   _____   _____
   _____   _____
   _____   _____
   _____   _____
   _____   _____
   _____   _____
   _____

13. List the basic and procedure-specific supplies that will be needed for the procedure.

   Pack _____
   Basin _____
   Gloves _____
   Blades _____
   Drapes _____
   _____
   Drains _____
   Dressings _____
   _____

   Suture – Type of Suture, Needle (if applicable), and Anticipated Tissue Usage

   _____   _____
   _____   _____
   _____   _____
   _____   _____
   _____   _____

   Pharmaceuticals

   _____   _____
   _____   _____
   _____   _____
   _____   _____

Miscellaneous

   _____   _____
   _____   _____
   _____   _____
   _____   _____
   _____   _____
   _____

14. Operative preparation: _____
   _____
   _____
   _____
   _____
   _____
   _____
   _____

15. What type of anesthesia will likely be used? Why?
   _____
   _____
   _____
   _____
   _____

16. List any special anesthesia equipment that may be needed. _____
   _____
   _____
   _____
   _____
   _____
   _____

17. Patient position during the procedure: _____
   _____
   _____
   _____
   _____

18. What supplies will be necessary for positioning?
    _____
    _____
    _____
    _____
    _____

19. What type of shave/skin preparation will be necessary (if any)? _____
    _____
    _____
    _____
    _____

20. Define the anatomic perimeters of the prep.
    _____
    _____
    _____
    _____
    _____

21. List the order in which the drapes will be applied, and describe any specific variations.
    _____
    _____
    _____
    _____
    _____
    _____
    _____

22. List any practical considerations.
    _____
    _____
    _____
    _____
    _____
    _____

23. List the procedural steps, and describe the preparatory and supportive actions of the STSR during each step (use additional space if necessary).

Operative Procedure	Technical Considerations
1.	•
	•
2.	•
	•
3.	•
	•
4.	•
	•
5.	•
	•

CHAPTER 17

Operative Procedure *continued*	Technical Considerations *continued*
6.	•
	•
7.	•
	•
8.	•
	•
9.	•
	•
10.	•
	•

24. What is the postoperative diagnosis? _____

25. Describe the immediate postoperative care.

26. What is the patient's long-term prognosis?

27. What are the possible complications? _____

28. Comments or questions: _____

29. What is the most valuable information you obtained from preparing this surgical procedure case study? _____

Case Studies

☐ CASE STUDY 1

Patricia has been experiencing several seemingly unrelated symptoms that include weight loss, headache, "heartburn," sweating, trembling, rapid heart rate, heat intolerance, and a feeling of anxiousness. Patricia's daughter finally convinced her to see her primary care physician, who has determined that Patricia has a tumor of the adrenal medulla.

1. What diagnostic studies are needed to confirm the diagnosis?

   _____
   _____
   _____
   _____

2. What is the name of Patricia's tumor, and how serious is it? Why?

   _____
   _____
   _____
   _____

3. What is the necessary treatment for Patricia's condition? What type of procedure will most likely be performed?

   _____
   _____
   _____
   _____

CASE STUDY 2

Six-year-old Belinda has been suffering from chronic urinary tract infections. The appearance of blood in her urine led to further testing that produced a diagnosis of PKD. Belinda's condition has nearly destroyed both kidneys. Belinda, her parents, and her twin sister, Melinda, are all extremely concerned about Belinda's future.

1. What does PKD mean, and from what type of PKD does Belinda suffer? _____

2. What does the term "parenchyma" mean? What are the parenchymatous organs? _____

3. Was invasive testing necessary to determine Belinda's diagnosis? _____

4. What course is the disease expected to follow? _____

5. What will be the most likely outcome for Belinda? _____

Orthopedic Surgery

CHAPTER 18

OBJECTIVES

After studying this chapter, the reader should be able to:

A 1. Discuss the relevant anatomy and physiology of the musculoskeletal system.

P 2. Describe the pathology of the musculoskeletal system that prompts surgical intervention and the related terminology.

3. Discuss any special preoperative orthopedic diagnostic procedures/tests.

O 4. Discuss any special preoperative preparation related to orthopedic procedures.

5. Identify the names and uses of orthopedic instruments, supplies, and drugs.

6. Identify the names and uses of special equipment related to orthopedic procedures.

7. Discuss the intraoperative preparation of the patient undergoing an orthopedic procedure.

8. Define and give an overview of the orthopedic procedure.

9. Discuss the purpose and expected outcomes of the orthopedic procedure.

10. Discuss the immediate postoperative care and possible complications of the orthopedic procedure.

S 11. Discuss any specific variations related to the preoperative, intraoperative, and postoperative care of the orthopedic patient.

Key Terms

Define the following:

1. Abduct _____

2. A.C. Joint _____

3. Adduct _____

4. -algia _____

5. Amphiarthrosis _____

6. Cancellous Bone _____

7. Cartilage _____

8. Comminuted _____

9. Compound Fracture _____

10. Cortical Bone _____

11. Diarthrosis _____

12. Epiphysis _____

13. Flexion _____

14. Greenstick Fracture _____

15. Ligament _____

16. Marrow _____

17. Osteogenesis _____

18. Osteomalacia _____

19. Pedicle _____

20. Proximal _____

21. Shoulder Joint _____

22. Splint _____

23. Synovium _____

24. Tendinitis _____

25. Valgus _____

Exercise A – Anatomy

1. Identify the skeletal bones shown in Figure 18-1.

   A. _____
   B. _____
   C. _____
   D. _____
   E. _____
   F. _____
   G. _____
   H. _____
   I. _____
   J. _____
   K. _____
   L. _____
   M. _____
   N. _____
   O. _____
   P. _____
   Q. _____
   R. _____
   S. _____
   T. _____
   U. _____
   V. _____
   W. _____
   X. _____
   Y. _____
   Z. _____
   AA. _____
   BB. _____

Figure 18-1

246　CHAPTER 18

Figure 18-2

Figure 18-3

2. Identify the structures of the vertebral column shown in Figure 18-2.

A. _____

B. _____

C. _____

D. _____

E. _____

F. _____

G. _____

H. _____

I. _____

J. _____

K. _____

L. _____

M. _____

N. _____

Orthopedic Surgery 247

3. Identify the vertebral structures shown in Figure 18-3.

   A. _____
   B. _____
   C. _____
   D. _____
   E. _____
   F. _____
   G. _____
   H. _____

4. Identify the structures shown in Figure 18-4.

   A. _____
   B. _____
   C. _____
   D. _____
   E. _____
   F. _____

5. Identify the bones of the pelvic girdle shown in Figure 18-5.

   A. _____
   B. _____

Figure 18-5

   C. _____
   D. _____
   E. _____
   F. _____
   G. _____
   H. _____
   I. _____
   J. _____
   K. _____

Figure 18-4

248   CHAPTER 18

Figure 18-6

6. Identify the elements of a long bone as shown in Figure 18-6.

A. _____

B. _____

C. _____

D. _____

E. _____

F. _____

G. _____

H. _____

I. _____

J. _____

K. _____

L. _____

M. _____

N. _____

O. _____

P. _____

7. List the five functions of the skeletal system.

   A. _____
   B. _____
   C. _____
   D. _____
   E. _____

8. List four factors that affect bone growth.

   A. _____
   B. _____
   C. _____
   D. _____

9. Define the term sesamoid, and give two examples of sesamoid bones. _____
   _____
   _____

   A. _____
   B. _____

10. What are the two main divisions of the skeleton? Briefly describe each division.

    A. _____
    _____
    B. _____
    _____

11. List the eight bones of the cranium.

    A. _____
    B. _____
    C. _____
    D. _____
    E. _____
    F. _____
    G. _____
    H. _____

12. Name the three bones that comprise the knee joint.

    A. _____
    B. _____
    C. _____

13. Describe the function of a gliding joint, and provide an example of a gliding joint. _____
    _____
    _____
    _____
    _____
    _____

14. Define circumduction, and give an example of a joint that is capable of circumduction. _____
    _____
    _____
    _____
    _____
    _____
    _____

15. In addition to calcium, name four other minerals that are stored within bone.

    A. _____
    B. _____
    C. _____
    D. _____

■ Exercise B – Pathology

1. What is ankylosis, and what is its cause? _____
   _____
   _____
   _____
   _____

2. How does vitamin D help to prevent osteomalacia? _____

3. Describe a greenstick fracture. _____

4. Does a patient suffering from subluxation have a fracture? Explain your answer. _____

5. Describe nonunion, and provide two reasons why nonunion may occur. _____

6. What is the cause of compartmental syndrome? How is compartmental syndrome manifested? _____

7. Why is the Lachman and Drawer examination performed? _____

8. What is the main complication of osteoporosis? _____

9. What bone is affected by a Colles' fracture? _____

10. A tumor of the cartilage is called a(n) _____.

11. What is the most common type of meniscal tear? Describe the defect. _____

12. _____ is an inflammation of the bone and bone marrow.

13. An elevated erythrocyte sedimentation rate (ESR) is an indicator of what type of condition? _____

14. What muscles comprise the rotator cuff? How will a tear of one or more of these muscles or their tendinous attachments affect the shoulder? _____

15. An arthrogram is an X-ray of what specific structure(s)? _____

■ Exercise C – Operation

1. What is meant by the term exsanguination? How does this apply to extremity surgery with the use of a tourniquet? _____

2. What is the maximum recommended time that tourniquet pressure may be applied to an upper extremity? Why? _____

3. What are two advantages to postoperative use of the CPM machine?

    A. _____

    B. _____

4. What precautions must be taken when the use of a C-arm is expected? _____

5. Describe the direction of the blade motion of a reciprocating saw. _____

6. What is bone wax, and how is it used? _____

7. List two situations in which a bone graft may be required.

    A. _____

    B. _____

8. What is the reason for application of irrigation fluid to the wound when sawing or drilling bone? _____

9. When using PMMA, what is the importance of using a closed mixing system? _____

10. What information must be documented following prosthesis insertion?

    A. _____

    B. _____

    C. _____

    D. _____

11. List two reasons why arthroscopy may be performed.

   A. _____

   B. _____

12. What is a reamer used to accomplish?

   _____

   _____

   _____

   _____

13. What are the three main advantages of maintaining laminar airflow in the OR during a surgical procedure?

   A. _____

   B. _____

   C. _____

14. Following closed reduction, what method of immobilization is commonly employed? _____

   _____

   _____

   _____

   _____

   _____

15. List the three types of traction.

   A. _____

   B. _____

   C. _____

ന# Exercise D – Specific Variations

Student Name _____ Date _____

Instructor _____

Surgical Procedure – Student Case Study Report

The student will be provided with basic patient information (real or simulated) and is expected to complete the following case study.

1. Procedure name: _____

2. Definition of procedure: _____

3. What is the purpose of the procedure? _____

4. What is the expected outcome of the procedure?

5. Patient age: _____

6. Gender: _____

7. Additional pertinent patient information: _____

8. Probable preoperative diagnosis: _____

9. How was the diagnosis determined? _____

10. Discuss the relevant anatomy. _____

11. List the general and procedure-specific equipment that will be needed for the procedure.

_____ _____
_____ _____
_____ _____
_____ _____
_____ _____

254 CHAPTER 18

12. List the general and procedure-specific instruments that will be needed for the procedure.

    _____   _____
    _____   _____
    _____   _____
    _____   _____
    _____   _____
    _____   _____

13. List the basic and procedure-specific supplies that will be needed for the procedure.

    Pack _____

    Basin _____

    Gloves _____

    Blades _____

    Drapes _____

    _____

    Drains _____

    Dressings _____

    _____

    Suture – Type of Suture, Needle (if applicable), and Anticipated Tissue Usage

    _____   _____
    _____   _____
    _____   _____
    _____   _____
    _____   _____

    Pharmaceuticals

    _____   _____
    _____   _____
    _____   _____
    _____   _____

    Miscellaneous

    _____   _____
    _____   _____
    _____   _____
    _____   _____
    _____   _____
    _____   _____

14. Operative preparation: _____
    _____
    _____
    _____
    _____
    _____
    _____
    _____

15. What type of anesthesia will likely be used? Why?
    _____
    _____
    _____
    _____
    _____
    _____

16. List any special anesthesia equipment that may be needed. _____
    _____
    _____
    _____
    _____
    _____
    _____
    _____

17. Patient position during the procedure: _____
    _____
    _____
    _____
    _____

18. What supplies will be necessary for positioning?
   _____
   _____
   _____
   _____
   _____

19. What type of shave/skin preparation will be necessary (if any)? _____
   _____
   _____
   _____
   _____
   _____

20. Define the anatomic perimeters of the prep.
   _____
   _____
   _____
   _____
   _____
   _____

21. List the order in which the drapes will be applied, and describe any specific variations.
   _____
   _____
   _____
   _____
   _____
   _____
   _____

22. List any practical considerations.
   _____
   _____
   _____
   _____
   _____
   _____
   _____

23. List the procedural steps, and describe the preparatory and supportive actions of the STSR during each step (use additional space if necessary).

Operative Procedure	Technical Considerations
1.	•
	•
2.	•
	•
3.	•
	•
4.	•
	•
5.	•
	•

256 CHAPTER 18

Operative Procedure *continued*	Technical Considerations *continued*
6.	•
	•
7.	•
	•
8.	•
	•
9.	•
	•
10.	•
	•

24. What is the postoperative diagnosis? _____
_____
_____
_____
_____
_____

25. Describe the immediate postoperative care.
_____
_____
_____
_____
_____
_____

26. What is the patient's long-term prognosis?
_____
_____
_____
_____
_____

27. What are the possible complications? _____
_____
_____
_____
_____
_____
_____

28. Comments or questions: _____
_____
_____
_____
_____
_____
_____

29. What is the most valuable information you obtained from preparing this surgical procedure case study? _____
_____
_____
_____

Case Studies

CASE STUDY 1

Ellenor is a 65-year-old female who was admitted to the hospital for a total hip arthroplasty.

1. Describe a routine draping procedure for this case. _____
   _____
   _____
   _____
   _____
   _____

2. What kind of incision is used? _____
   _____
   _____
   _____
   _____
   _____

3. After the femoral osteotomy guide is placed over the lateral femur and neck, what should the STSR plan to do next? _____
   _____
   _____
   _____
   _____
   _____

4. Will the incision be drained? _____
   _____
   _____
   _____
   _____
   _____

5. Describe the immediate postoperative care the patient will receive. _____
   _____
   _____
   _____
   _____
   _____

CASE STUDY 2

Leroy was admitted to the emergency department with a fracture of the left tibia and fibula. The fracture was reduced, the leg placed in a cast, and Leroy was sent home.

1. Why are casts placed on limbs with reduced fractures? _____

2. What is the meaning of the term "distraction"? Why is it a problem? _____

3. What is the most important factor in bone healing? _____

4. To what does the term "delayed union" refer? _____

Cardiothoracic Surgery

CHAPTER 19

OBJECTIVES

After studying this chapter, the reader should be able to:

A 1. Discuss the relevant anatomy of the cardiovascular and respiratory systems.

P 2. Describe the pathology that prompts cardiac or thoracic surgical intervention and the related terminology.

3. Discuss any special preoperative diagnostic procedures/tests for the patient undergoing cardiac or thoracic surgery.

O 4. Discuss any special preoperative preparation procedures.

5. Identify the names and uses of cardiovascular and thoracic instruments, supplies, and drugs.

6. Identify the names and uses of special equipment for the cardiac or thoracic procedure.

7. Discuss the intraoperative preparation of the patient undergoing a cardiac or thoracic procedure.

8. Define and give an overview of the cardiac or thoracic procedure.

9. Discuss the purpose and expected outcomes of the cardiac or thoracic procedure.

10. Discuss the immediate postoperative care and possible complications of the cardiac or thoracic procedure.

S 11. Discuss any specific variations related to the preoperative, intraoperative, and postoperative care of the patient undergoing a cardiac or thoracic procedure.

Key Terms

Define the following:

1. Alveoli _____
2. Aneurysm _____
3. Arrhythmia _____
4. Atria _____
5. Bradycardia _____
6. Cardiac Cycle _____
7. Ductus Arteriosus _____
8. Hyaline Cartilage _____
9. Infarction _____
10. Infiltrate _____
11. Mediastinum _____
12. Myocardium _____
13. Oxygenated _____
14. Pericardium _____
15. Plaque _____
16. Pleura _____
17. Prolapse _____
18. PVC _____
19. Regurgitation _____
20. Stent _____
21. Systole _____
22. Tachycardia _____
23. Tamponade _____
24. Thoracic Duct _____
25. Ventricles _____

Cardiothoracic Surgery   261

■ Exercise A – Anatomy

1. Identify the structures of the thorax shown in Figure 19-1.

   A. _____
   B. _____
   C. _____
   D. _____
   E. _____

Figure 19-1

2. Identify the structures shown in Figure 19-2.

   A. _____
   B. _____
   C. _____
   D. _____
   E. _____
   F. _____
   G. _____
   H. _____
   I. _____
   J. _____

Figure 19-2

262 CHAPTER 19

K. _____
L. _____
M. _____
N. _____
O. _____
P. _____
Q. _____
R. _____
S. _____

3. Identify the structures of the heart and the great vessels shown in Figure 19-3.

A. _____
B. _____
C. _____
D. _____
E. _____
F. _____
G. _____

H. _____
I. _____
J. _____
K. _____
L. _____
M. _____
N. _____
O. _____
P. _____
Q. _____
R. _____
S. _____
T. _____
U. _____
V. _____
W. _____
X. _____
Y. _____

Figure 19-3

Cardiothoracic Surgery 263

G. _____
H. _____
I. _____
J. _____
K. _____

5. Identify the cardiac valves shown in Figure 19-5.

A. _____
B. _____
C. _____

6. Identify the structures shown in Figure 19-6.

A. _____
B. _____
C. _____
D. _____
E. _____
F. _____
G. _____
H. _____
I. _____
J. _____
K. _____
L. _____
M. _____
N. _____
O. _____

Figure 19-4

4. Identify the structures shown in Figure 19-4.

A. _____
B. _____
C. _____
D. _____
E. _____
F. _____

Figure 19-5

Figure 19-6

264   CHAPTER 19

7. List the following events in the proper chronological sequence to complete the cardiac cycle.

   A. _____ Atria contract

   B. _____ AV node stimulated

   C. _____ Impulse moves through right and left bundle branches

   D. _____ Impulse transmitted to bundle of His

   E. _____ Impulse travels via internodal atrial pathways

   F. _____ Purkinje fibers stimulated

   G. _____ SA node generates initial impulse

   H. _____ Ventricles contract

8. Trace the flow of blood from the time it leaves the venae cavae to the time it enters the aorta by placing the following elements in the correct order.

   A. _____ Aorta

   B. _____ Aortic valve

   C. _____ Bicuspid valve

   D. _____ Left atrium

   E. _____ Left ventricle

   F. _____ Lungs

   G. _____ Pulmonary arteries

   H. _____ Pulmonary valve

   I. _____ Pulmonary veins

   J. _____ Right atrium

   K. _____ Right ventricle

   L. _____ Tricuspid valve

   M. _____ Venae cavae

9. Name the three layers of the heart wall.

   A. _____

   B. _____

   C. _____

10. Name the four cardiac valves and describe their locations.

    A. _____
    _____

    B. _____
    _____

    C. _____
    _____

    D. _____
    _____

11. Define cardiac output. _____
    _____
    _____
    _____
    _____

12. What is the function of the bundle of His?
    _____
    _____
    _____
    _____

13. Name and describe the two layers of the pleura.

    A. _____
    _____

    B. _____
    _____

14. What structures are contained within the mediastinum? _____
    _____
    _____
    _____
    _____

15. Name the principal muscles of inspiration.

    A. _____

    B. _____

Exercise B – Pathology

1. List three methods used to detect lung tumors.

   A. _____

   B. _____

   C. _____

2. Describe the condition known as flail chest.
   _____
   _____
   _____
   _____

3. Penetrating chest trauma will result in which condition? What treatment is necessary? _____
   _____
   _____
   _____
   _____

4. What is cardiac tamponade? What treatment is necessary? _____
   _____
   _____
   _____
   _____

5. List the three types of thoracic outlet syndrome and the cause of each.

   A. _____
   _____

   B. _____
   _____

   C. _____
   _____

6. Describe a Type II dissecting aneurysm of the thoracic aorta. What does dissecting mean in reference to an aneurysm? _____
   _____
   _____
   _____

7. What is the composition of an atheroma? What causes formation of an atheroma? _____
   _____
   _____
   _____
   _____
   _____

8. Which cardiac enzyme levels rise following myocardial infarction?

   A. _____

   B. _____

   C. _____

9. List three complications of myocardial infarction.

   A. _____

   B. _____

   C. _____

10. What effect does alcohol have on cardiac tissue?
    _____
    _____
    _____
    _____

11. Describe the condition known as patent ductus arteriosus, list the symptoms, and provide treatment options. _____
    _____
    _____
    _____
    _____
    _____

12. List the four cardiac defects seen in the classic form of tetralogy of Fallot.

    A. _____

    B. _____

    C. _____

    D. _____

13. List two variable and two inherited risk factors for coronary atherosclerosis.

    A. _____

    B. _____

    C. _____

    D. _____

14. What is/are the cause(s) of mitral regurgitation? _____

15. A commissurotomy is performed to treat which condition? _____

Exercise C – Operation

1. List the two types of mediastinoscopy, and provide a brief description of each.

    A. _____

    B. _____

2. Is bronchoscopy strictly a diagnostic procedure? Explain your answer. _____

3. In which position will the patient be placed in order to accomplish a posterolateral thoracotomy? _____

4. Explain the difference between lobectomy and pneumonectomy. _____

5. What is the purpose of inserting a double-lumen endotracheal tube during a thoracotomy? _____

6. In which position will the patient be placed to accomplish a median sternotomy? _____

7. What is empyema? What procedure is performed to treat empyema? _____

8. Which body functions are taken over by the pump oxygenator during open-heart surgery? _____

9. Describe the placement of the cannulas necessary for a cardiopulmonary bypass. _____

_____

_____

_____

10. Name two blood vessels that are most commonly used as the graft during CABG procedures.

    A. _____

    B. _____

11. List the two basic types of materials that are used for cardiac valve replacement.

    A. _____

    B. _____

12. What are the two main components of a pacemaker?

    A. _____

    B. _____

13. Why is it important to have an open-heart team on "standby" during PTCA? _____

_____

_____

_____

14. Is cardiopulmonary bypass necessary for closure of a patent ductus arteriosus in an infant?

_____

_____

_____

_____

15. What is the purpose of administering potassium cardioplegia solution during open-heart procedures? _____

_____

_____

_____

CHAPTER 19

■ Exercise D – Specific Variations

Student Name _____ Date _____

Instructor _____

Surgical Procedure – Student Case Study Report

The student will be provided with basic patient information (real or simulated) and is expected to complete the following case study.

1. Procedure name: _____
   _____
   _____

2. Definition of procedure: _____
   _____
   _____
   _____
   _____

3. What is the purpose of the procedure? _____
   _____
   _____
   _____
   _____

4. What is the expected outcome of the procedure?
   _____
   _____
   _____
   _____

5. Patient age: _____

6. Gender: _____

7. Additional pertinent patient information: _____
   _____
   _____

8. Probable preoperative diagnosis: _____
   _____
   _____
   _____
   _____
   _____

9. How was the diagnosis determined? _____
   _____
   _____
   _____
   _____

10. Discuss the relevant anatomy. _____
    _____
    _____
    _____
    _____
    _____
    _____

11. List the general and procedure-specific equipment that will be needed for the procedure.

    _____   _____
    _____   _____
    _____   _____
    _____   _____
    _____   _____

12. List the general and procedure-specific instruments that will be needed for the procedure.

    _____ _____
    _____ _____
    _____ _____
    _____ _____
    _____ _____
    _____

13. List the basic and procedure-specific supplies that will be needed for the procedure.

    Pack _____

    Basin _____

    Gloves _____

    Blades _____

    Drapes _____
    _____

    Drains _____

    Dressings _____
    _____

    Suture – Type of Suture, Needle (if applicable), and Anticipated Tissue Usage

    _____ _____
    _____ _____
    _____ _____
    _____ _____
    _____ _____
    _____ _____

    Pharmaceuticals

    _____ _____
    _____ _____
    _____ _____
    _____ _____

Miscellaneous

_____ _____
_____ _____
_____ _____
_____ _____
_____ _____
_____ _____

14. Operative preparation: _____
    _____
    _____
    _____
    _____
    _____
    _____
    _____

15. What type of anesthesia will likely be used? Why?
    _____
    _____
    _____
    _____
    _____

16. List any special anesthesia equipment that may be needed. _____
    _____
    _____
    _____
    _____
    _____
    _____

17. Patient position during the procedure: _____
    _____
    _____
    _____

270   CHAPTER 19

18. What supplies will be necessary for positioning?
_____
_____
_____
_____
_____

19. What type of shave/skin preparation will be necessary (if any)? _____
_____
_____
_____
_____
_____

20. Define the anatomic perimeters of the prep.
_____
_____
_____
_____
_____

21. List the order in which the drapes will be applied, and describe any specific variations.
_____
_____
_____
_____
_____
_____

22. List any practical considerations.
_____
_____
_____
_____
_____

23. List the procedural steps, and describe the preparatory and supportive actions of the STSR during each step (use additional space if necessary).

Operative Procedure	Technical Considerations
1.	•
	•
2.	•
	•
3.	•
	•
4.	•
	•
5.	•
	•

Cardiothoracic Surgery 271

Operative Procedure continued	**Technical Considerations** continued
6.	•
	•
7.	•
	•
8.	•
	•
9.	•
	•
10.	•
	•

24. What is the postoperative diagnosis? _____

25. Describe the immediate postoperative care.

26. What is the patient's long-term prognosis?

27. What are the possible complications? _____

28. Comments or questions: _____

29. What is the most valuable information you obtained from preparing this surgical procedure case study? _____

Case Studies

☐ CASE STUDY 1

Elroy has been transported to the emergency department following a motor vehicle accident (MVA). He was the unrestrained driver of one of the vehicles, and his body hit the steering wheel on impact. Elroy has dyspnea, tachypnea, and tachycardia, appears extremely anxious, and is showing signs of shock. Upon examination, the emergency physician notes distant heart sounds, hypotension, and jugular venous distension. A Swan-Ganz catheter placed by the physician reveals equal RA and pulmonary capillary wedge pressures and an elevated CVP.

1. What type of injury is suspected as a result of the blunt chest trauma? _____

2. What diagnostic exams are indicated? _____

3. What is the treatment for this condition? _____

CASE STUDY 2

Timothy, a 49-year-old construction worker, fell from a scaffold and was rushed to the emergency department, where he was evaluated by the trauma team. Timothy complained of chest pain, and severe respiratory distress was noted by the physician. Chest X-ray revealed fractures of the 5th and 6th ribs on the right and absence of lung markings over the affected area.

1. In addition to Timothy's fractured ribs, what other condition is affecting him? _____

2. What treatment will be provided? _____

3. What type of wound drainage system will be needed? Why? _____

4. Will a wound dressing be necessary? If so, what type and why? _____

Peripheral Vascular Surgery

CHAPTER 20

OBJECTIVES

After studying this chapter, the reader should be able to:

A 1. Discuss the relevant anatomy of the peripheral vascular system.

P 2. Describe the pathology that prompts surgical intervention of the peripheral vascular system and the related terminology.

3. Discuss any special preoperative peripheral vascular diagnostic procedures.

O 4. Discuss any special preoperative preparation procedures.

5. Identify the names and uses of peripheral vascular instruments, supplies, and drugs.

6. Identify the names and uses of special equipment.

7. Discuss the intraoperative preparation of the patient undergoing the peripheral vascular procedure.

8. Define and give an overview of the peripheral vascular procedure.

9. Discuss the purpose and expected outcomes of the peripheral vascular procedure.

10. Discuss the immediate postoperative care and possible complications of the peripheral vascular procedure.

S 11. Discuss any specific variations related to the preoperative, intraoperative, and postoperative care of the patient undergoing peripheral vascular surgery.

CHAPTER 20

■ Key Terms

Define the following:

1. Adventitia _____
_____

2. Bifurcation _____
_____

3. Capillary _____
_____

4. Claudication _____
_____

5. Contralateral _____
_____

6. Diastolic _____
_____

7. Dissecting (as pertains to aneurysm) _____
_____

8. Embolus _____
_____

9. Fogarty Catheter _____
_____

10. In Situ _____
_____

11. Innominate _____
_____

12. Intima _____
_____

13. Ischemia _____
_____

14. Mitigate _____
_____

15. Morbidity _____
_____

16. Mortality _____
_____

17. Occlude _____
_____

18. Papaverine _____
_____

19. Patent _____
_____

20. Phrenic _____
_____

21. Pledget _____
_____

22. Plethysmography _____
_____

23. Sinus _____
_____

24. Thrombus _____
_____

25. Valve _____
_____

■ Exercise A – Anatomy

1. Identify the branches of the aorta shown in Figure 20-1.

   A. _____
   B. _____
   C. _____
   D. _____
   E. _____
   F. _____
   G. _____
   H. _____
   I. _____

Peripheral Vascular Surgery 277

T. _____

U. _____

2. Identify the systemic arteries shown in Figure 20-2.

A. _____

B. _____

C. _____

D. _____

E. _____

F. _____

G. _____

H. _____

Figure 20-1

J. _____

K. _____

L. _____

M. _____

N. _____

O. _____

P. _____

Q. _____

R. _____

S. _____

Figure 20-2

278   CHAPTER 20

I. _____
J. _____
K. _____
L. _____
M. _____
N. _____
O. _____
P. _____
Q. _____
R. _____
S. _____
T. _____
U. _____
V. _____
W. _____
X. _____
Y. _____
Z. _____
AA. _____
BB. _____
CC. _____
DD. _____
EE. _____
FF. _____
GG. _____
HH. _____

3. Identify the systemic veins shown in Figure 20-3.

A. _____
B. _____
C. _____
D. _____
E. _____

Figure 20-3

F. _____
G. _____
H. _____
I. _____
J. _____
K. _____
L. _____

M. _____

N. _____

O. _____

P. _____

Q. _____

R. _____

S. _____

T. _____

U. _____

V. _____

W. _____

X. _____

Y. _____

Z. _____

4. Identify the structures of the blood vessels shown in Figure 20-4.

A. _____

B. _____

C. _____

D. _____

E. _____

F. _____

G. _____

H. _____

I. _____

5. List the three tunics of a blood vessel wall, and briefly describe the composition and function of each structure.

A. _____

B. _____

C. _____

Figure 20-4

6. What structures receive arterial blood from the brachiocephalic artery? _____

_____

_____

_____

_____

7. Which artery or arteries, if any, branch off the ascending aorta? _____

_____

_____

_____

8. Each common carotid artery bifurcates into two sections. Provide the names of the two branches and the structures supplied with arterial blood from each.

   A. _____

   B. _____

9. What effect does the autonomic nervous system have on vasoconstriction? _____

10. Which is larger, the lumen of an artery or the lumen of a vein in a similar location? _____

11. What effect does vasodilation have on the blood pressure? _____

12. What is blood pressure? _____

13. List three factors that affect arterial blood pressure.

    A. _____

    B. _____

    C. _____

14. What does the term "resistance" describe within the cardiovascular system? How does increased resistance affect blood pressure? _____

15. List the three main branches of the common hepatic artery, and name the structure(s) served by each.

    A. _____

    B. _____

    C. _____

Exercise B – Pathology

1. What causes claudication? _____

2. List the four signs/symptoms of acute arterial occlusion.

   A. _____

   B. _____

   C. _____

   D. _____

3. There are several types of emboli. Name two.

   A. _____

   B. _____

4. List three types of treatment for embolism.

   A. _____

   B. _____

   C. _____

5. What is the shape of a fusiform aneurysm? What portion of the aorta is most often involved?

6. Varicose veins commonly involve the saphenous vein. Describe the condition, and list two possible treatments.

7. What term is used to describe inflammation of a vein?

8. What is the cause of a TIA (transient ischemic attack)?

9. What is plaque?

10. What examinations may be performed to identify a lesion of the common carotid artery?

11. What is the difference between ischemia and necrosis?

12. What are the signs/symptoms associated with a TIA?

13. List four risk factors associated with the development of peripheral vascular disease.

   A.
   B.
   C.
   D.

14. How is the establishment of collateral blood flow encouraged in patients with vascular insufficiency of the lower extremity?

15. List three physical signs of vascular insufficiency of the lower extremity.

   A.
   B.
   C.

Exercise C – Operation

1. In what situation will contrast solution (e.g., Conray, Hypaque) be needed on the sterile field?

2. List three hemostatic agents that are typically used during peripheral vascular surgical procedures.

    A.

    B.

    C.

3. What is a Fogarty catheter used to accomplish?

4. What is the purpose of an intraluminal stent?

5. Vascular grafts are available in several configurations. Name two.

    A.

    B.

6. Why do some types of vascular graft material have rigid rings (exoskeleton) built into the graft? In which location are the reinforced grafts commonly implanted?

7. What is the primary indication for carotid endarterectomy?

8. During carotid endarterectomy, is the use of a shunt necessary? Why?

9. Vascular grafts are available in several materials. Name two.

    A.

    B.

10. What instruments are typically used to perform an arteriotomy?

11. What is the purpose of creating a tunnel during a femoral popliteal bypass?

12. List two complications that may arise following implantation of a composite graft.

    A.

    B.

13. Why is it necessary to pre-clot a vascular graft that is made of knitted polyester? _____

14. What is a patch suture? How is it prepared?

15. Why is it important for the STSR to remain sterile and keep the back table and Mayo stand intact until the patient has been transported to the PACU? _____

Exercise D – Specific Variations

Student Name _____ Date _____

Instructor _____

Surgical Procedure – Student Case Study Report

The student will be provided with basic patient information (real or simulated) and is expected to complete the following case study.

1. Procedure name: _____
   _____
   _____

2. Definition of procedure: _____
   _____
   _____
   _____

3. What is the purpose of the procedure? _____
   _____
   _____
   _____

4. What is the expected outcome of the procedure?
   _____
   _____
   _____

5. Patient age: _____

6. Gender: _____

7. Additional pertinent patient information: _____
   _____
   _____

8. Probable preoperative diagnosis: _____
   _____
   _____
   _____
   _____

9. How was the diagnosis determined? _____
   _____
   _____
   _____
   _____

10. Discuss the relevant anatomy. _____
    _____
    _____
    _____
    _____
    _____

11. List the general and procedure-specific equipment that will be needed for the procedure.

    _____ _____
    _____ _____
    _____ _____
    _____ _____
    _____ _____

12. List the general and procedure-specific instruments that will be needed for the procedure.

   _____ _____
   _____ _____
   _____ _____
   _____ _____
   _____ _____
   _____

13. List the basic and procedure-specific supplies that will be needed for the procedure.

   Pack _____

   Basin _____

   Gloves _____

   Blades _____

   Drapes _____

   _____

   Drains _____

   Dressings _____

   _____

   Suture – Type of Suture, Needle (if applicable), and Anticipated Tissue Usage

   _____ _____
   _____ _____
   _____ _____
   _____ _____
   _____ _____

   Pharmaceuticals

   _____ _____
   _____ _____
   _____ _____
   _____ _____

Miscellaneous

   _____ _____
   _____ _____
   _____ _____
   _____ _____
   _____ _____
   _____ _____

14. Operative preparation: _____

   _____
   _____
   _____
   _____
   _____
   _____
   _____

15. What type of anesthesia will likely be used? Why?

   _____
   _____
   _____
   _____
   _____
   _____

16. List any special anesthesia equipment that may be needed. _____

   _____
   _____
   _____
   _____
   _____
   _____
   _____

17. Patient position during the procedure: _____

   _____
   _____
   _____
   _____

CHAPTER 20

18. What supplies will be necessary for positioning? _____

19. What type of shave/skin preparation will be necessary (if any)? _____

20. Define the anatomic perimeters of the prep. _____

21. List the order in which the drapes will be applied, and describe any specific variations. _____

22. List any practical considerations. _____

23. List the procedural steps, and describe the preparatory and supportive actions of the STSR during each step (use additional space if necessary).

Operative Procedure	Technical Considerations
1.	•
	•
2.	•
	•
3.	•
	•
4.	•
	•
5.	•
	•

Operative Procedure *continued*	Technical Considerations *continued*
6.	•
	•
7.	•
	•
8.	•
	•
9.	•
	•
10.	•
	•

24. What is the postoperative diagnosis? _____

25. Describe the immediate postoperative care.

26. What is the patient's long-term prognosis?

27. What are the possible complications? _____

28. Comments or questions: _____

29. What is the most valuable information you obtained from preparing this surgical procedure case study? _____

Case Studies

CASE STUDY 1

Joe is a 50-year-old male who was brought to the emergency department in hemorrhagic shock due to a ruptured abdominal aneurysm. The surgeon called the surgery department to alert them that he is in transit with the patient for immediate intervention. The OR team leader, in turn, has notified the STSR and circulator who are assigned to the case. The surgical team springs into action.

1. What supplies will the STSR open onto the sterile field first? _____

2. What instrument sets will be needed? _____

3. What instruments will be needed first? _____

☐ CASE STUDY 2

Wayne, a 67-year-old male, presented to the emergency department with the following symptoms: severe hypertension, malaise, orthopnea, peripheral edema, and decreased urinary output. He is a pack-a-day smoker and is grossly overweight.

1. What is the preliminary diagnosis? _____

2. What diagnostic examination is considered the gold standard for confirmation of the preliminary diagnosis? _____

3. Will surgical intervention be necessary? If so, what procedure will be scheduled? _____

CHAPTER 21

Neurosurgery

OBJECTIVES

After studying this chapter, the reader should be able to:

A 1. Discuss the relevant anatomy and physiology of the neurological system.

P 2. Describe the pathology that prompts surgical intervention of the neurological system and the related terminology.

3. Discuss any special preoperative neurological diagnostic procedures/tests.

O 4. Discuss any special preoperative preparation procedures related to neurosurgery.

5. Identify the names and uses of neurosurgical instruments, supplies, and drugs.

6. Identify the names and uses of special equipment related to neurosurgery.

7. Discuss the intraoperative preparation of the patient undergoing the neurosurgical procedure.

8. Define and give an overview of the neurosurgical procedure.

9. Discuss the purpose and expected outcomes of the neurosurgical procedure.

10. Discuss the immediate postoperative care and possible complications of the neurosurgical procedure.

S 11. Discuss any specific variations related to the preoperative, intraoperative, and postoperative care of the neurosurgical patient.

CHAPTER 21

■ Key Terms

Define the following:

1. Abscess _____

2. Acute _____

3. Autonomic Nervous System _____

4. Caudal _____

5. Cerebellum _____

6. Cerebrum _____

7. Circle of Willis _____

8. CNS _____

9. Decompress _____

10. Dysraphism _____

11. Epidural _____

12. Extruded _____

13. Glioma _____

14. Hematoma _____

15. ICP _____

16. Integration _____

17. Meninges _____

18. Osteophyte _____

19. Parasympathetic _____

20. PNS _____

21. Radiculopathy _____

22. Somatic Nervous System _____

23. Sympathetic _____

24. TIA _____

25. Transphenoidal _____

Exercise A – Anatomy

1. Identify the major divisions of the autonomic nervous system shown in Figure 21-1.

   A. _____
   B. _____
   C. _____
   D. _____
   E. _____
   F. _____
   G. _____
   H. _____
   I. _____
   J. _____
   K. _____

2. Identify the structures of the external surface of the brain shown in Figure 21-2.

   A. _____
   B. _____
   C. _____
   D. _____
   E. _____
   F. _____
   G. _____
   H. _____
   I. _____
   J. _____
   K. _____

Figure 21-1

Figure 21-2

294   CHAPTER 21

Figure 21-3

4. Identify the cranial nerves shown in Figure 21-4.

A. _____
B. _____
C. _____
D. _____
E. _____
F. _____
G. _____
H. _____
I. _____
J. _____
K. _____
L. _____
M. _____

3. Identify the meninges and related structures shown in Figure 21-3.

A. _____
B. _____
C. _____
D. _____
E. _____
F. _____
G. _____
H. _____
I. _____
J. _____
K. _____
L. _____

Figure 21-4

Figure 21-5

5. Identify the ventricles of the brain and related structures shown in Figure 21-5.

A. _____

B. _____

C. _____

D. _____

E. _____

F. _____

G. _____

H. _____

I. _____

J. _____

K. _____

L. _____

296   CHAPTER 21

Dorsal

Figure 21-6

6. Identify the pathway of impulses (reflex arc) and related structures shown in Figure 21-6.

   A. _____
   B. _____
   C. _____
   D. _____
   E. _____
   F. _____
   G. _____
   H. _____
   I. _____
   J. _____
   K. _____
   L. _____
   M. _____
   N. _____
   O. _____

7. Name the eight bones of the cranium.

   A. _____
   B. _____
   C. _____
   D. _____
   E. _____
   F. _____
   G. _____
   H. _____

8. Name the three meningeal layers in sequence from outermost to innermost.

   A. _____
   B. _____
   C. _____

9. Where is CSF formed? How is it formed? _____
   _____
   _____
   _____
   _____

10. Name the three branches of the trigeminal nerve, and describe the functions of the target tissue(s) innervated by each branch.

    A. _____
       _____
    B. _____
       _____
    C. _____
       _____

11. What are the three primary functions of the nervous system?

    A. _____
       _____
    B. _____
       _____
    C. _____
       _____

12. What are the two subdivisions of the ANS, and what is the basic function of each division?

    A. _____
       _____
    B. _____
       _____

13. What is the circle of Willis? _____
    _____
    _____
    _____

14. The auditory processing area of the brain is located in the _____ lobe of the brain.

15. The vital centers of the brain (respiratory, cardiac, vasomotor) are contained in which portion of the brain stem? _____
    _____
    _____
    _____
    _____

Exercise B – Pathology

1. Hydrocephalus has several causes. List three.

   A. _____
   B. _____
   C. _____

2. List three types of obstruction of the aqueducts between the ventricles that can lead to hydrocephalus.

   A. _____
   B. _____
   C. _____

3. Describe the condition known as spondylosis.
   _____
   _____
   _____
   _____
   _____

4. Name two radiographic techniques that may be used to identify spinal disorders, and describe how each is used.

   A. _____
      _____
   B. _____
      _____

CHAPTER 21

5. What is the difference between a subdural hematoma and an epidural hematoma? _____
   _____
   _____
   _____
   _____

6. Define craniosynostosis, and describe the method(s) for diagnosing the condition. _____
   _____
   _____
   _____
   _____

7. Describe spina bifida. _____
   _____
   _____
   _____
   _____

8. List the three classifications (locations) of spinal cord tumors and the symptoms of each.

   A. _____
   _____

   B. _____
   _____

   C. _____
   _____

9. Carpal tunnel syndrome affects which nerve at what level? _____
   _____
   _____
   _____
   _____

10. What is the underlying cause of growth hormone (GH) overproduction? _____
    _____
    _____

_____
_____

11. Describe two symptoms that a patient with herniated nucleus pulposus may experience.

    A. _____

    B. _____

12. What is the most common type of brain tumor?
    _____
    _____
    _____
    _____

13. What symptoms are associated with acoustic neuroma? Which nerve is affected? _____
    _____
    _____
    _____
    _____

14. The condition known as tic douloureux is also known as _____ _____. What surgical procedure is performed to relieve the symptoms of tic douloureux? _____
    _____
    _____
    _____
    _____

15. List and describe the three types of subdural hematoma.

    A. _____
    _____

    B. _____
    _____

    C. _____
    _____

Exercise C – Operation

1. What is the Mayfield pin-fixation device used to accomplish? _____

2. How do Raney clips differ from aneurysm clips? _____

3. Access to the occipital lobe of the brain may be accomplished with the patient in either of two positions. Name the two possible positions.

    A. _____

    B. _____

4. What supplies may be necessary to remove scalp hair in the operating room? _____

5. List three options for treatment of a cerebral aneurysm.

    A. _____

    B. _____

    C. _____

6. It is important to restrict movement in and around the sterile field at all times, but why is this especially true during procedures near the cerebellopontine angle? _____

7. List the four main components of the ventriculoperitoneal shunt.

    A. _____

    B. _____

    C. _____

    D. _____

8. Name two approaches that can be used for surgery of the pituitary.

    A. _____

    B. _____

9. List two materials that can be implanted during cranioplasty and that can be molded to fit the cranial defect.

    A. _____

    B. _____

10. List two methods by which the bone flap is secured to the cranium following a craniotomy.

    A. _____

    B. _____

11. Why are two separate Mayo stands needed for transphenoidal procedures? _____

12. What is papaverine used for during arterial intracranial surgery? _____

13. What is the ideal temperature for irrigation fluid that will be used intracranially? _____

14. What is the CUSA, and how is it used?

15. What is ICP? How is it monitored?

■ Exercise D – Specific Variations

Student Name _____ Date _____

Instructor _____

Surgical Procedure – Student Case Study Report

The student will be provided with basic patient information (real or simulated) and is expected to complete the following case study.

1. Procedure name: _____
   _____
   _____

2. Definition of procedure: _____
   _____
   _____
   _____
   _____

3. What is the purpose of the procedure? _____
   _____
   _____
   _____
   _____

4. What is the expected outcome of the procedure?
   _____
   _____
   _____
   _____

5. Patient age: _____

6. Gender: _____

7. Additional pertinent patient information: _____
   _____
   _____
   _____

8. Probable preoperative diagnosis: _____
   _____
   _____
   _____
   _____
   _____

9. How was the diagnosis determined? _____
   _____
   _____
   _____
   _____

10. Discuss the relevant anatomy. _____
    _____
    _____
    _____
    _____
    _____

11. List the general and procedure-specific equipment that will be needed for the procedure.

    _____   _____
    _____   _____
    _____   _____
    _____   _____
    _____   _____

12. List the general and procedure-specific instruments that will be needed for the procedure.

    _____ _____
    _____ _____
    _____ _____
    _____ _____
    _____ _____
    _____ _____

13. List the basic and procedure-specific supplies that will be needed for the procedure.

    Pack _____

    Basin _____

    Gloves _____

    Blades _____

    Drapes _____
    _____

    Drains _____

    Dressings _____
    _____

    Suture – Type of Suture, Needle (if applicable), and Anticipated Tissue Usage

    _____ _____
    _____ _____
    _____ _____
    _____ _____
    _____ _____
    _____ _____

    Pharmaceuticals

    _____ _____
    _____ _____
    _____ _____
    _____ _____

Miscellaneous

_____ _____
_____ _____
_____ _____
_____ _____
_____ _____
_____ _____

14. Operative preparation: _____
    _____
    _____
    _____
    _____
    _____
    _____
    _____

15. What type of anesthesia will likely be used? Why?
    _____
    _____
    _____
    _____
    _____
    _____

16. List any special anesthesia equipment that may be needed. _____
    _____
    _____
    _____
    _____
    _____
    _____

17. Patient position during the procedure: _____
    _____
    _____
    _____
    _____

18. What supplies will be necessary for positioning?

    _____
    _____
    _____
    _____
    _____

19. What type of shave/skin preparation will be necessary (if any)? _____

    _____
    _____
    _____
    _____
    _____

20. Define the anatomic perimeters of the prep.

    _____
    _____
    _____
    _____
    _____

21. List the order in which the drapes will be applied, and describe any specific variations.

    _____
    _____
    _____
    _____
    _____
    _____
    _____
    _____

22. List any practical considerations.

    _____
    _____
    _____
    _____
    _____
    _____

23. List the procedural steps, and describe the preparatory and supportive actions of the STSR during each step (use additional space if necessary).

Operative Procedure	Technical Considerations
1.	•
	•
2.	•
	•
3.	•
	•
4.	•
	•
5.	•
	•

Operative Procedure *continued*	Technical Considerations *continued*
6.	•
	•
7.	•
	•
8.	•
	•
9.	•
	•
10.	•
	•

24. What is the postoperative diagnosis? _____

_____

_____

_____

_____

25. Describe the immediate postoperative care.

_____

_____

_____

_____

_____

26. What is the patient's long-term prognosis?

_____

_____

_____

_____

27. What are the possible complications? _____

_____

_____

_____

_____

_____

28. Comments or questions: _____

_____

_____

_____

_____

_____

29. What is the most valuable information you obtained from preparing this surgical procedure case study? _____

_____

_____

_____

Case Studies

☐ CASE STUDY 1

Dr. Roberts was summoned to the emergency department to see a 34-year-old male who was brought in complaining of a severe headache of sudden onset. The patient described the headache as "violent, bursting, and explosive." He stated that it was the worst headache that he has ever experienced. The patient is nauseous, photophobic, and complaining of pain in the lower back. A lumbar puncture revealed blood within the cerebrospinal fluid.

1. What is the preliminary diagnosis? _____

2. In addition to the lumbar puncture, what other diagnostic tests should be performed? _____

3. What diagnostic test is considered the gold standard for this condition? _____

4. What are the treatment options? _____

CASE STUDY 2

Jamma, a 43-year-old secretary for a law firm, presents to Dr. Michaels with complaints of numbness, tingling, and pain in the right hand. Dr. Michaels notes during the examination that the symptoms are localized to the thumb, index finger, long finger, and medial aspect of the ring finger. He also notes that pain occasionally radiates up the arm into the shoulder. Jamma states that the pain awakens her at night.

1. What is the diagnosis? _____

2. What is the etiology of the syndrome? _____

3. How is the condition treated? List the conservative and surgical options. _____